No More Hair Drama

No More Hair Drama

By: Antoinette Shar'ron Johnson

Order this book online at www.trafford.com
or email orders@trafford.com

Most Trafford titles are also available at major online book retailers.

© Copyright 2010 Antoinette Shar'ron Johnson.
All rights reserved. No part of this publication may be reproduced, stored in a retrieval
system, or transmitted, in any form or by any means, electronic, mechanical, photocopying,
recording, or otherwise, without the written prior permission of the author.

Printed in Victoria, BC, Canada.

ISBN: 978-1-4269-0717-3 (Soft)

*We at Trafford believe that it is the responsibility of us all, as both individuals
and corporations, to make choices that are environmentally and socially sound.
You, in turn, are supporting this responsible conduct each time you purchase a
Trafford book, or make use of our publishing services. To find out how you are
helping, please visit www.trafford.com/responsiblepublishing.html*

*Our mission is to efficiently provide the world's finest, most comprehensive
book publishing service, enabling every author to experience success.
To find out how to publish your book, your way, and have it available
worldwide, visit us online at www.trafford.com*

Trafford rev. 01/13/2010

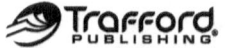 www.trafford.com

North America & international
toll-free: 1 888 232 4444 (USA & Canada)
phone: 250 383 6864 ♦ fax: 812 355 4082 ♦ email: info@trafford.com

Dedication

I started to write this book after I locked my hair on December 26, 2001, as a response, from my perspective, concerning how African hair textures are viewed. Also, I wanted to address some of my own personal issues related to hair drama in order to paint a picture of what we as women of African descent have gone through concerning our hair through the years.

I dedicate this book to my mother, Patricia Wilson, and to the memory of my grandmother, Hilda Mae Harrell, for all their love, strength, selflessness, courage, and for being so positive throughout the years. You gave me above and beyond 100% of yourselves and that I could never repay. I do not have enough words that would suffice for all that you have given to me. Thank you for being my inspiration!

I dedicate this book to all the African American women who are wondering, contemplating, procrastinating, or pondering about what next to do with your hair. This book is for the women who are looking for a spiritual awakening and freedom from struggling with what next to do with your hair. This book is dedicated to those women who are worried about what others will think of them when seen for the first time with their new hairstyle should you choose to go natural. This book is dedicated to the women who are struggling with their identity and are looking for a solution in the search of finding themselves. This book is dedicated to the women who are tired of seeing more hair in the comb than on their head. This book is for the women who are tired of living their lives according to someone else's perspective of beauty. This book is also for the women who are adventurous and looking for something new and exciting. Whether you are looking to relax, curl, weave, press, lock, braid, wear a wig or short afro, just be sure of your reasons for doing so and feel good about yourself no matter what. Ultimately, you have to be comfortable with you in whatever you choose.

Women must come together to be strong in all that is accomplished. In keeping God first, we can do all things. Remember that the prayers of the righteous do indeed avail much. Our prayers are a direct channel to God, and through our communication, his spirit will then transcend upon us. Continue to be an inspiration to others and let your light shine upon the world. In whatever you do, remember that we are one and should continue to be each other's strength and listening ear. I am my sister's keeper, which is one of the reasons why I decided to write this book and share my experiences with you.

Table of Contents

Acknowledgments

Since this is my first book, I felt it only fitting to acknowledge the many people who have given me love and support not only for this project but also throughout my life.

First, I would like to give honor to God who is the head of my life. You are my alpha and omega—my beginning and my end. I thank you and love you Jesus for your courage, strength, endurance, and your constant ability to love unconditionally. I will love, worship, and praise you always!

To my husband, Maury: You are a part of the road I call destiny. My puzzle would not be complete if you were not in it. Thank you for your love, support, sense of humor, strength, and friendship through thick and thin. I love you from the breadth and depth of my soul.

To my daughter, Jasmyne: My ladybug. You are such a blessing to be around, you are a loving person, and you have such a beautiful spirit. I am very proud of you. I thank God for you always. I love you dearly!

To my son, Maury II: My little sweetheart. I thank God for you because of your ability to make me laugh. Thank you for having such a wonderful sense of humor, a sensitive spirit, and for being as thoughtful as you are toward others. I love you dearly!

To my mom, Patricia Wilson: Thank you for choosing to give me life and always supporting my every endeavor. You are the light at the end of my tunnel, my "Rock of Gibraltar," and my source of inspiration. I will always remember your encouraging words and your tenacity. I love you very much.

To my dad, Clifton Wilson: Thank you for always being the knight in shinning armor in our lives. My mom was truly blessed when you came into her life and swept her off her feet. I love you for being everything that a dad should strive to be.

To my dad, John Kearse: I hope that you find the peace in your life that you deserve, and I hope that you find that positive path in your life. God bless! I love you.

To Nanny, the late Mrs. Hilda Mae Harrell: My heart and soul cries out to you, and I thank you for gracing me with your existence. I am eternally grateful to you for your wisdom, goodness, and unconditional love for us. You have given to many people. I love you forever. We shall see each other again!

To Granddad, Mr. Sidney Harrell: Thank you for the many years of being in my life. Also, thank you for the day you met Miss Hilda Mae Brown for if it were not for your meeting I would not be here. I love you always.

To Grandma and Grandpa Kearse and the Kearse family: I am thankful to have you all in my life and wish that we would have seen each other more often as I was growing up. I hope that our relationship can grow to greater heights.

To my sister, Sharise: I remember the day mom and dad brought you home from the hospital. I was so proud to be your big sister. You are one of the wisest and most intelligent people that I know. I am thankful to you for your listening ear and positive spirit. God bless your marriage, children, and to all that are connected to you. I love you always.

To my brother-in-law, Jeff: Thank you Jeff for coming to Sharise's rescue! You are truly a gem. I love you.

To my sister, Violet: You are meant to do great things. Believe in yourself always as your family and God does. You have an incredible amount of strength. I know life can be a struggle, but we can always rely and trust in God for our strength. Always remember that.

To my dad, Curtis and step-mom, Shirley Clark: I am glad to have had the opportunity to meet you, and I hope this relationship will continue to grow. Now the puzzle is complete!

To my sister, Lashiem: What a blessing it was to find you. I am grateful that God has given me another sister. I hope one day that we can share many memories!

To my sister, Tiffaney: I truly hope that you allow God to direct your path in life. Only He can do it. I wish you many, many blessings.

To my sister and brother, Erica and Henry: It was wonderful meeting you. I wish the very best for you and your families. Remember to keep striving for the best that life has to offer you.

To my sister, Jennifer: The Lord has blessed you with Jaliyah, Jamaze, and Jiaya. I wish the best for you and that you always remain positive in life. God Bless you.

To my brother, Timothy: I know we have not been close for the majority of our lives, but that does not mean that I have not thought about you through the years. I wish you lots of happiness in your life. God Bless.

To the Wilson family: I am pleased to have met all of you. You made me feel welcome and a part of your family from the beginning, and I thank you for that. God bless you always!

To Aunt Carol and Uncle Charlie: Thank you for the fun parties that you have had through the years. No one does it quite like you! I pray God continues to bless you!

To Carla (Bunnie): Thanks for the years of fun, laughs, and great conversation. I also thank you for adopting Brandi and giving her a loving home!

To my second mom, Mildred Johnson: Thank you for your kind spirit and for treating me like one of your own children. You are truly one in a million and an amazing person! I love you.

To Juanita Vaughn: I am thankful to you for babysitting me and for being a part of my life. You have touched me in a big way in this life.

To Darlis Johnson: You are a great friend and sister. You have made me laugh for many years. I am convinced that laughter cures all. Thanks for the laughter!

To Dionne Johnson-Clark: You are truly inspirational holding a household down with five children yet you still smile. Thank you for being you!

To Shon Clark: I pray that God gives you strength and guidance in life. Just lean on Him, and He will provide you with what you need.

To Columbus and Deirdre Johnson: I hope that God almighty directs your path and orders your steps where He wants you to go. Lean on Him and He will guide you.

To Walter Johnson: You have been truly blessed in your life. Your comedic talents are second to none. Always keep your sense of humor. It is truly therapeutic.

To Tierra Woodson: You are such a great person. Continue to move toward your dreams, and do not let anything stop you from achieving them.

To Maurice Johnson: I pray that God shines his light on you and gives you strength throughout your life.

To Denise & Gerry Beckles: Your wisdom and spirit-filled lives are a wonderful testimony to many. I cannot tell you how much you have touched me with your loving spirit. Thank you for availing yourselves to me in my times of need.

To Jesse and Vickie Crawford: Thank you for being there for me and for listening to me when I was going through. You have an awesome spirit! You are truly blessed and I love your energy and ability to be there for many people.

To the late Walter Carrington: I thank you for your kindness toward me while you were here. God bless you.

To Lena Carrington: You have such a warm spirit that is so inviting, and it transcends to everyone you meet. You have treated me like one of your own children and I really appreciate that about you. Thank you for your spirit.

To the late Levi and Bobbie Lee Johnson: You have always made me feel like a part of the family. I treasure you for your union because if it were not for you I would never have met my husband.

To the rest of the Johnson family: Thank you for welcoming me with open arms!

To my nieces and nephews: I pray that your lives are richly blessed with all that God has to offer you. Remember that education is truly the key to a successful life. Stay strong and focused in all that you do.

To my cousins: I thank God for my extended family you all are the greatest!

Special thanks to all of my other family members who may not be mentioned by name. Thank you for affecting my life in one way or another!

To my friend, Alisa Douglas: Well, what can I say to a friendship three decades long! You are as crazy now as you were back in the day. Keep your sense of humor in tact. You are definitely one of a kind! God Bless you always! Love ya!

To my friend, Lorri Smith: One of my closest and dearest friends in this world. You are like a sister to me. We can spend months without talking or seeing one another and when we do talk and see each other again it is as if the conversation never ended. Thank you for being such a bright spirit and positive influence in my life! Love ya, girl!

To my friend, Brigid Orozco: You have a lot to be proud of in your life. I feel very blessed to have known you for so long and impressed by the fact that you have done an amazing job with your daughter. Your husband and daughter are blessed to have you. Keep traveling on the path to progress. Love always.

To my friend, Eloise (Dee Dee) Jacobs: You helped me to see the vision, helped me have the confidence, and supported me as I embarked upon this hair locking adventure. I will never forget your encouragement and friendship. I thank you from the bottom of my heart!

To my friends, Robert and Jacky Barnett: Your marriage is one to be admired. I think you are such a selfless couple in all that you have done for others, and I am thankful that you have entered into my life.

To my friends, Roy and Dian Stevens: You are a fun and outstanding couple. I am truly grateful to know you. I feel very inspired and encouraged by you and the strength you display in difficult situations. Thank you for being a part of my life!

To my friends, Sabrina and David Cole: The two of you have been very inspirational in my life. I appreciate our conversations and the Christian life that the two of you lead. You are a great example for your children.

To my friend, Linda Jackson: I am so thankful that our daughters met. It has been great getting to know you, and I look forward to many years of friendship with you. God Bless you always!

To my friend, Avis Roper: It is wonderful to have met such kind people as you and your husband, David. I am thankful that our daughters are friends. I am grateful to God for His allowing me to be exposed to positive people.

To the members of Girl Scout Troop 7595: It has certainly been a lot of fun being involved with you ladies and the fabulous group of girls since the year 2000. I hope God continues to Bless you and your families.

To all of my other friends: You know who you are. Thanks for the love!

Special thanks to: Pastor Hooper (for allowing me to start the Mount Zion Newsline and to write articles on behalf of Mount Zion), First Lady Pam Hooper, and my Mount Zion A.M.E. family for all of your love, prayers, friendship, and support!

To Marvetta Troop: Thank you for helping me with launching my writing career. I truly thank you for all that I have learned from you.

Thanks To my friends at UMDNJ: Lynn Boettinger, Juana Canela, Susan Giordano, Lois Grau, Susan Hammerman, Thelma Hitchman, Annette Madison, Margaret Mitchell, Hanaan Osman, Dolores Rivera, Renee Rogers, Stephanie Spencer Valentin, Natalie Trump, Markeeta Watts, Maudie Woods, and David Wright.

To Ramat, my original lock hairstylist: Thank you for starting me on my way to the world of hair locking on December 26, 2001.

To Alyssa Caldwell, my new hairstylist: It was truly a blessing to find you, thanks to Dee Dee Jacobs. Your hairstyling gifts and talents are next to your positive spirit. I wish all the best for you and your family.

To my journalism instructor, Mr. Glenn Townes: My thanks to you for lending your writing experience to me and showing me the "ins and outs" of the world of journalism. You are a gem!

To the Rutgers Women's Basketball Team: I commend you because you are beautiful from the inside out and the way you conduct yourselves shows how eloquent you are. I applaud and respect you for your courage, strength, and determination in light of the recent controversy. I pray the Lord God Almighty always shows you favor in your lives in all that you do.

To my cover designer, Vanessa Brantley-Newton: I do not believe anything happens by coincidence or accident. We met at the right time, in the right place, and under the right circumstances. I believe God ordained it. God Bless you in all your endeavors.

Special thanks to all of my survey participants for your honest answers and the time you dedicated to the survey!

Special thanks to my book review group: Linda Bright, Eloise Jacobs, Annabelle Johnson, Yvonne Johnson, Sharise Keels, Lorri Smith, and Dian Stevens for your candidness and dedication to this project.

Special, special thanks to my creative consultant Miss Jasmyne G. Johnson.

This book is in memory of those who have departed this life before the publishing of this book. God bless you always!

Preface

This is a non-fiction book about the roads that women travel in the world of hair. The book is designed to be a fun learning tool for women who may be at a crossroads in their lives concerning their hair and are looking into different options for preserving and maintaining their hair. This book is highly based upon many women's experiences but is a true testament of the African American woman's journey into the pursuit of the perfect and ideal style. This book will take you on a journey through the many different styles, times, and attitudes toward the directions that African American women and women of African descent have taken concerning their hair. This book will definitely be a trip down memory lane for many women.

I started to write this book after I locked my hair on December 26, 2001. My mission was to tell a story about my plight in finding myself through my hair, being comfortable in my skin, loving my distinct African features, and truly loving who God made me to be. I realized that through the years and my many hairstyles that I was on the "search" for something. However, I was looking for something that was already there. I was beautiful and did not realize it. I got tired of my self-esteem and pride being tied into my hair or in what others thought of me.

It is my estimation that women of African descent continually connect hair with self-esteem and self-worth to the degree that we look at extremes – if our hair is "nappy or kinky" then it is bad, and if our hair is "straight" or "loosely curled" then it is good. I placed a challenge on myself not to be caught up in what others deem appropriate for me, and I am placing that same challenge on you. You decide for yourself what is appropriate for you. Think outside of the box!

This book was also written to inspire women to do what they feel is necessary for themselves, create dialogue, reflect upon the negatives and positives in life, help to gain an understanding of self, and uplift women throughout the journey of different hair processes. This book was also designed to help women to be able to choose whatever style works best for them and provides a look into – the negative and positive drama that goes into the African American woman's hair care journey!

Introduction

Women of African descent have worn their hair micro-braided, kinky twisted, two-strand twisted, coiled, cornrowed, afro'd, locked, pressed, weaved, wig'd, fingerwaved, multi-colored, afro puffed, layered, bobbed, French Rolled, Senegalese Twisted, Jheri Curled, razor cut, tipped, teased, pageboy'd, permed, bouffanted, pixie'd, natural, ponytailed, punked, spiked, Shirley Temple curled, wrapped, doobied, blunt cut, French Twisted, frosted, textured, crimped, fishtail plaited, flat twisted, sister locked, and silky locked. You name it women of African descent have done it and have been at the forefront of setting trends in hair styling throughout the years all over the world.

While conducting the research for this project, I discovered that women have dealt with a lot of stress in attaining the perfect coif. In our desperation, at times, we have allowed ourselves to be talked into many styles that were no good for our hair. African American women take their hair very seriously. A lot of their identity is wrapped in their hair looking perfect. When African American women go to the beauty parlor, they hope that the men in their lives would like the style that they chose. When women ask men, "How is my hair?" the response may be "it's alright" which can be disappointing to many women because they thought the style was perfect. What is it about the style that causes such an unexcited or unfavorable response? Is it natural vs. chemical or vice versa? Is it the style itself? The hair survey, as you will see in Chapter 7, had some very interesting responses from the men which addressed the "How is my hair?" question and other issues concerning their wives or girlfriend's hair.

Women feel pressure when trying to stay presentable. We know that the coif is one of the most important things about the African American woman's makeup. If the hair is not right, then some women do not feel right. So much goes into a woman's appearance and a lot of thought is placed into putting that ultimate look together. At times, women want to be adventurous with their hair, but that is not always accepted in some places like the corporate arena. The corporate atmosphere does not always allow for too much deviation from the "norm" -- the norm being straightened hair. However, if women do not want the straightened hair look then they should wear their hair as they choose and understand that in some arenas they may have a difficult time because of the politics that could exist. Some African American women tend to do what others feel more comfortable with rather than what they desire to do for themselves. Subsequently, women of African descent have been very compromising throughout the years. African American women should consider doing what is in their best interest instead of what others want for them.

Women like Madame C.J. Walker helped to revolutionize the hair care industry and modern day beauty salons. She was one of the pioneers who helped beauticians of today become as creative as they have become over the years. More and more I am discovering that we need to go back to the basic professionalism that was taught during the time when Madame C.J. Walker and "Beauty Culture" school was around. Women were treated with the respect and dignity that they deserved.

How we treat ourselves is a very important aspect of maintaining healthy hair. Having a healthy mind, body, and soul directly contributes to having healthy hair. We need to understand that the mind, body, and soul need to be unified in order to aid in our overall body function. In connection with the mind, body, and soul, having high self-esteem allows you to make the appropriate choices for you. There are times when you will be expected to "fit in" to what the "status quo" wants, but it is not worth losing yourself in the process. Dealing with people can sometimes be very difficult in our daily walk, and people cannot allow negative situations to occupy space in their minds.

In this life, people endure both positive and negative situations that affect their self-esteem. Although African American women can be best friends, they can be worst enemies too by buying into such concepts as "good hair" and "bad hair. What that means is if your hair is of a wavy, shiny, straight grade naturally then it is considered good and if it is of a kinky, dull, coarse grade then it is considered bad. African American women have to be supportive of one another and speak more positively concerning hairstyle choices. My experiences with women have been both positive and negative. On the positive side, my grandmother and mother have been great influences because of their strength, high self-esteem, and supportiveness of me in my hair choices. On the negative side, I have dealt with women who have made negative comments to me about my current hairstyle (locks). My mother always said that I had "the best hair" because anything could be done to it. That, to me, sounds like I had "good hair." Even though my hair was very thick and "kinky" she still considered my hair to be the best.

At the early stages of my hair drama, I can remember having my hair done in cornrows braided into a Mohawk-style. I also remember having cornrows and beads at age 11, a Vigorol® relaxer at age 12, the curl during the ages of 13-18, another relaxer from ages 19-22, the curl from ages 22-23 (which was a complete nightmare because it was blown dry and my hair proceeded to fall out in clumps). Next, I went natural, I had another try at the curl (after cutting all of my hair off to start over), and back to the relaxer, then braids, another try at the relaxer, more braids, and the natural again, and finally locks. My hair has gone through the war. Around 1980, I got my first curl done by a family member. It was one of those boxed kits. I begged my mother to get a curl, and she consented. I had a lot of hair at this point and after I got the curl, my hair never grew back to the same thickness that it was before I got the curl. All these experiences caused me to feel like I was on a hair drama merry-go-round and never getting off! Throughout these experiences, in addition to expressing my creativity, I was searching for the best hairstyle that works for me and my hair type. The journey has been both positive and negative.

During my journey into finding the hairstyle that suits me best, I realized that I had some trying experiences with many beauticians. From dealing with unreasonable wait times, listening to foul language, and sitting in unclean establishments, I have truly only had two good experiences that come to mind which I will elaborate on in Chapter 5 which is about the Hair Care Industry. I hope that people have more good experiences than bad ones at the beauty parlors and barbershops that they frequent.

Join me in exploring the many aspects of what we face as women—the drama. Although we look at "drama" as being a negative, it can actually provide a balance between the positive and negative things and is essential to life. It is a collaboration of our experiences and a testament of the ability to endure all things.

Chapter 1

In the Beginning...
Understanding Our Past

Madame C.J. Walker was an incredible woman with great foresight. Born Sarah Breedlove, December 23, 1867, she was creative, innovative, and a definite genius. She created a hair care system for African American women back in the early 1900's to aid in achieving healthy hair and hair growth. During the 1890's she had a scalp condition that caused her to lose her hair. To correct the hair loss, she created a product that consisted of a home remedy and products made by an entrepreneur named Annie Malone. The combination of these products helped her hair to grow back and in better condition than before. At this point, she decided to market her product in order to help other African American women achieve similar results.

The Walker System, as it was called, consisted of a shampoo, a scalp conditioning and healing ointment also called pomade, and a hot comb in order to press out hair that was very curly or kinky. Before her system came into existence, African American women would press out their hair with an iron on a flat surface in order to make it more manageable and less kinky. She took the product on the road and began selling it in the Northern and Southern states. The product also became very popular in Europe. Through her efforts, she became the first African American woman to become a self-made millionaire! Not only did she market the Walker System, she patented a permanent wave machine, which curled both black and white women's hair and created long lasting wavy hairstyles.

In 1908, she opened the Walker College of Hair Culture (what is known today as a School of Cosmetology) in Pittsburgh, PA, to train her hair care sales team known as "Walker Agents." In addition to her hair care products, she sold a line of cosmetics in order to allow women the ability to enhance their beauty that helped to boost their self-confidence. She offered meaningful employment to her licensed Walker Agents. Her business was not just a place of employment but also a place where women felt empowered and experienced a personal growth through their hard work.

Madame C.J. Walker was a philanthropist and also a social activist for women's rights issues. Much of her fortune she generously donated to African American organizations. The employees were encouraged by her to support African American organizations and the African American community. She worked diligently in her business and other efforts until her death on May 25, 1919. Madame C.J. Walker was truly a role model for African American women and exemplified success in all that she did. She proved to us that as long as we persevere we could achieve many things in life.

Growing up with a Grandmother who was a Beautician

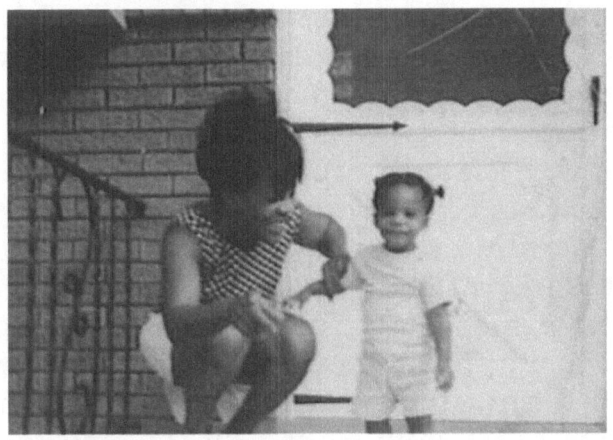

My grandmother (Nanny as my siblings and I called her) was a phenomenal woman. She used to talk about how she graduated from "Beauty Culture School" and became a licensed beautician. She was extremely proud of that accomplishment, and rightfully so. Nanny learned how to care for hair with administering proper shampooing and conditioning techniques, press and curl, permanent hair coloring, styling, etc. You name it she could do it with ease.

One of the best experiences I had with her is the time I spent at her house on Saturday mornings getting my weekly beauty treatment. Nanny would start me with a good shampoo and conditioning treatment then dry my hair under the big dome hair dryer or let it air dry. She would then have me sit in my "special chair" in the kitchen and drape a towel around me. The "kitchen beauty parlor" seemed to be tradition in many African American homes back then, and the kitchen was a gathering place in which African American people did a lot of socializing. To this day, people still gather in the kitchen to socialize.

While getting my hair done, I never felt any pain when she combed through it because she took great ease in caring for my hair. I do not know how she did my hair with the amount of patience she had because my hair was extremely thick. All I can think of is that she really loved doing hair not to mention that she loved me. After all, I was her first grandchild! I distinctly remember the smell of Dax Pressing Oil® and the hot comb on the stove like it was yesterday. Prior to starting the pressing process, she would get out some heavy-duty equipment that included the straightening comb (two different sizes small and large) and for special occasions the curling iron. The entire process went like this...she would take the pressing oil, place a bit on the back of her hand, and then rub some of it through my hair. After that, she would comb through my hair and section it.

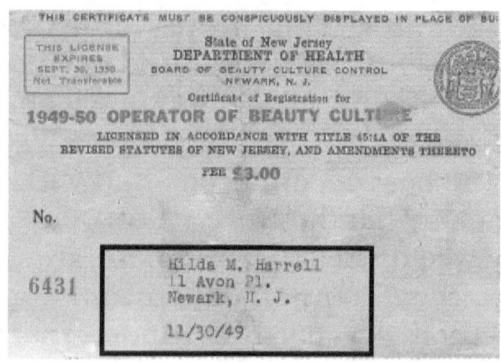

Next, the pressing comb went on top of the burner on the stove. After that, the straightening comb would be applied through my hair from root to end. I felt a cool breeze, as she would blow in order to cool down the hot comb as it went through my hair. Nanny had an old towel sitting on the counter so that she could wipe off residue from the comb before placing it back on the burner after she had run the comb through my hair. She would do this section by section until my whole head was complete. Finally, she would run the comb through my entire head one more time just to make sure that all of my hair was pressed thoroughly.

The part that always made me cringe was when she had to press out the edges (in the front) and the "kitchen" (the area of hair at the nape of the neck). That is when she took out the small-sized comb. I cringed because I always anticipated being burned. She would say, "Hold still" in a very patient and angelic voice. When she told me to hold still and I actually listened, I was never burned. The way that she turned my black, coarse, thick, dull hair into shiny and more manageable hair was nothing short of a miracle. After she was finished, she would put my hair into two or three ponytails, and off I went to play for the rest of my Saturday.

When I was having my hair pressed, it was much healthier compared to when I started having it chemically processed.

During those times when there was a special occasion like school picture taking or a dance recital, she would whip out that manual curling iron. One side of the iron was completely still the other side swung around and looked very complicated to use. I would watch her as she handled this curling iron.

She literally wrapped the contraption around her fingers (like a samurai warrior), took a section of hair, and with ease just pulled it through to curl my hair. I was completely amazed!

There were times when she would do my hair in stages. If she was in the middle of cooking dinner, then I had to wait until she was done. In that case, she would just wash my hair, dry it, and press it later. I remember vividly one day she dried my hair and told me to go outside and play for a while and she would call me in when she was finished with what she was doing. "O.K.," I said and scurried around to find something to put on my head. One of my friends from the neighborhood, saw me playing outside and came out to join me. She wanted to know why I was wearing the hat and before I could explain, she pulled my hat off, ran with it, and laughed hysterically. I swore that I looked like *Buck Wheat* from *The Little Rascals* and chased her diligently for that hat. I was so embarrassed and humiliated! Maybe I was embarrassed because of negative vibes that I picked up for having thick and coarse hair. Back then, women were moving away from the afro and started looking at other hairstyles including straight styles. I can laugh about the "Buck Wheat" incident now, but back then, it was no laughing matter!

At a certain point in her life, Nanny could no longer do hair due to arthritis that developed in her hands. I often wished that my daughter had had the privilege of getting her hair done by Nanny. We talked about life, and she shared stories about her growing up in Newark with her brothers, sisters, cousins, etc. It was not just about making me look fantastic because Nanny could hook my hair up; it was about the bonding that took place in Nanny's kitchen, and the time we shared was something that I will never forget. It was more than just getting my hair done. It was about us having a special relationship that I would cherish my whole life.

Chapter 2

Dedicated to My "Sistas" and Sisters

From the Past to the Present: Dealing with Negative Terms

African American women have grown up dealing with many negative terms. Terms like nappy-headed, knotty-headed, peasy-headed, picaninny, and Buck Wheat have been permanently etched into our memories from childhood and have permeated throughout the culture into adulthood. The term good hair is also a negative term. It sends the message that if you do not have long straight or wavy hair ("good hair") then you have "bad" hair. African American women have had to contend with these negative terms for too long. When I was growing up, I was very familiar with the term "good hair" from other African Americans because we felt bad about our hair. These thoughts originated from slavery time. African American's contend with these negative connotations to this day and the result of negativity can be very damaging.

What is good hair?

What is your definition of good hair? My definition of good hair is if I have hair on my head regardless of texture, then that is good. Many of us grew up in a time when people who had straight or wavy hair were considered to have "Indian" in their family. Truth be told, many of us wished we had "Indian" in our family back in the day when we were teased about our hair texture if it was considered to be "nappy." Our own peers within our race have brought on a lot of this animosity about our hair overtly. Many people were angry that they were given what they thought was "bad hair" and that anger transferred onto people that had the straighter texture hair, therefore, causing a dislike of the person in some way. Those girls with the straighter texture hair were accused of thinking they were "cute" when, in many cases, they were far from being conceited. That thought was fabricated out of insecurity on the part of the person with the less desirable hair texture.

There was a time when those thoughts of "good hair/bad hair" did a turnaround and African Americans found that there was power in their hair. That time was called "The Black Power Movement." At that time, African Americans did not want to straighten their hair because they wanted to make a statement. Afros were in style in the 1960's and cornrows and braids were starting to receive popularity in the 1970's and 1980's. The 1960's were turbulent times due to rioting, and African Americans were involved in the rebellion back then. The goal was to deviate from what the "white man" wanted and to receive the respect that was overdue. Back then, there were many problems concerning racial prejudice and not a substantial pick of the positions at companies that were considered "high level" even if you were college educated. African

Americans felt that their hair was one of the few things that they could control and that no one could tell them what to do with their hair. They were in control or so they thought.

After the movement, African Americans wanted to "fit in" again so they changed their hair to a more acceptable style--a straighter style comparable to those of our Caucasian counterparts to get a more "Europeanized" look. During that time, if an African American wanted a career in "Corporate America" they had better conform and straighten their hair instead of attempt to be "militant" by wearing natural styles.

Many African American's believe that their hair is not presentable in its natural state because of what they may have been told. Truthfully, many styles work well with natural hair such as braiding or locking. Today, those styles are beginning to become popular among women and men in American culture regardless of race. Many people think that locking and "dreadlocks" are one in the same. Locking has evolved from the Rastafarian Dreadlock. The techniques for both are slightly different. For more information on the Rastafarian Dreadlock, please see the bonus chapter at the end of the book in Appendix I.

We must realize that having hair is a blessing and the sheer fact that you have hair is GOOD. Many African American women are losing their hair for various reasons including Alopecia (a scalp condition in which permanent baldness occurs) and breakage due to different problems. Some women are allergic to the chemicals in relaxer creams. In addition, tight braiding can cause breakage and baldness.

Why do African Americans have so many hair struggles?

It starts from the beginning...your childhood. Why do little girls today feel that they NEED their hair relaxed? Peer pressure can be very devastating particularly to one's self-image. What you feel about yourself is quite important. You must have a positive mental attitude to overcome these negative situations. Try not to allow any negativity penetrate your spirit. Your self-image/worth is crucial to your health and well-being. If you maintain a good positive self-image then it will shine through physically and that includes your hair.

Much of this self-hatred began back during the times of slavery. Those slaves that had a more European look (skin tone and hair) received the preferential treatment, were able to make residence indoors, and were treated better than those who had very distinct African features. In addition, those who were able to "pass" for white were preferred over others.

African American women need to be more positive and uplifting toward one another. I remember someone referring to a woman's locked hair as "feeling like a rug" and this reference was made in front of a lot of people. People should not put others down and should think before they speak. Everyone should feel free to wear the style that he or she feels most comfortable. We have a long way to go because we are still tearing each other down. We should be more complimentary toward one another instead of negative. If a woman wants to lock, braid, relax or whatever, she needs the support of other women in whatever choice she decides to make. Many people make negative comments about another person's natural hair because they have been convinced that natural hair is not acceptable. They have been convinced that natural hair is not beautiful because it is coarse and not bone straight. We all should feel beautiful about ourselves regardless of what we choose to do with our hair.

One evening, I watched the television show America's Next Top Model. One of the models had her hair braided. She was told that she had to remove her braids because they are not "marketable." After that comment, I thought to myself, "What was meant by the term marketable, and who determines the market?" I believe consumers determine the market and keep the economy going. It makes absolutely no sense that a market is a determining factor in the hairstyle that someone chooses. Why does it seem that afro-textured hair or styles of an African origin are so threatening or problematic? She may have had a sentimental attachment to her braids because they were an extension of her self-worth and pride for being of African descent. It is tragic that African Americans feel that they are expected to continually compromise and define themselves through someone else's idea of what is beautiful. The ironic part of this whole expectation of compromise is that I have been seeing young Caucasian girls wearing historically Afrocentric styles like cornrows, braids, flat twists, etc. Is there an expectation for African Americans to compromise, still?

Turn a negative into a positive

The understanding is that by wearing our hair in a relaxed state, it is more acceptable by Corporate America and sometimes, our African American counterparts, but we have to learn to be comfortable with ourselves, and with our decisions. It took me a long time to be comfortable with my own features: full lips, hair, body type, etc. The older I get, the more I love what God has created me to be. As a result, I am no longer interested in impressing others. I will no longer live my life according to someone else's viewpoint of beauty! I determine what is beautiful to me.

Flipping the Script: A Caucasian Woman's Perspective on Hair

In an article written by Ashley Parrish entitled, *"The Long and Short of It,"* published on www.marieclaire.com, Ms. Parrish talks about her experience of going from having long hair to having short hair after eight years of having long, thick hair. She described the anguish that she went through as her hair was being chopped off. It was an emotional time for her as the beautician cut her hair.

What I discovered after reading this article was that women of different races tend to feel the same way as it pertains to hair. Some women cry in the chair, some women leave the hair salon half way done, and some women cry for days. Their hair is more than just hair. It has become an extension of them—a very important part of their lives. The hair may have been with them through some major life events like weddings, graduations, their first apartment, etc. which indicates an attachment.

After the initial shock of the hair cut, Ms. Parrish felt like a new woman. She felt brave, courageous, and vigorous. She stated that women go from being fearful to brave after getting a hair cut because they feel refreshed and brand new. She states, "For many women, our hair is part of our personalities," which is the reason why women are so emotional when they get their hair cut after having long hair for a number of years. The confidence that women get after getting their hair cut gives women a boost in their self-esteem.

For Ms. Parrish, she received double takes from people, and some people who knew her did not recognize her immediately. Although she missed her long hair at times, she does not know if she will grow her hair long again.

Although I understood the emotions involved when black women cut their hair, I had no idea that white women experienced the same emotions when having their haircut. After reading this article, I now realize that women of different races have a spiritual connection with their hair.

Chapter 3

Mind, Body, and Soul

In order to function from a healthy perspective, the mind, body, and soul must be synchronized. This means that we have to maintain the health of our mind by feeding it knowledge, maintain the health of our body by feeding it nourishing food, and maintain the health of our soul by feeding it spirituality. We should maintain ourselves in many ways, i.e. positive attitude, exercise, eating a balanced diet, relationship with God through prayer, meditation, reading self-empowerment books, etc. Good conversation and fellowship with people also helps us to be healthy in the mind, body, and soul.

There are times in life when we have to confront negative situations and we must learn to deal with them as best as we can. How we handle these situations are determined by how healthy we are in the mind, body and soul. It has been said that laughter is the best medicine for a healthy mind and body because it is a great way to relieve stress.

So what does all of this have to do with hair? Truthfully, you can do some damage to your hair if your mind, body, and soul are out of balance. For example, I knew of someone at the workplace who was under terrible stress and pressure and that situation caused her to lose her hair in large amounts daily. The stress caused her to be out of balance in her mind, body, and soul. I also had problems with hair loss. Not handling stress properly coupled with having my hair chemically processed, was a recipe for disaster for me. The hair in the back of my head came out and it looked as though my hair had been cut when it actually had not. This I called my unscheduled haircut.

The Mind Aspect – Positive Mental Health

In our society, it is particularly difficult to stay positive in this negative world. Truthfully, the more you try to stay positive the more negative forces attempt to weigh you down. Our mind is the driving force for every move and decision that we make. If you are over burdened with negativity in your life, focusing can be a difficult thing to achieve. Too much stress and not releasing that stress properly can cause you to have deteriorating health which could result in hair problems. Some of the key components to maintaining a healthy mind are calming your mind by releasing stress through positive thought, exercising your brain in daily thinking, reading, listening to relaxing music, meditating, etc.

Worry and fear can be detrimental to one's mental health, thereby affecting one's overall health. By being caught up in a cycle of worry and fear, you can cripple yourself and lose control. I will elaborate more on this in the "The Soul Aspect" section of this chapter.

Deep breathing aids in combating fatigue helps to provide revitalization of the mind. Oxygen is necessary to aid in proper brain functioning.

The Body Aspect – Good Physical Health

The statement "You are what you eat" is very true. Good health is crucial to having not only a healthy body but also healthy hair. Remember the saying, "You are what you eat." Eating foods that contain plenty of vitamins, minerals, and protein is important in order to maintain the body. You can find the food pyramid at www.mypyramid.gov for more information on proper eating. Subsequently, since the hair comes from the body, the vitamins that you ingest will be absorbed by the cells that create the hair aiding in healthier hair. In addition, different types of medications, lack of proper nutrition, and vitamin deficiencies can cause hair loss.

Starting your day with breakfast to begin the daily cycle of proper nutrition is very important. Studies have shown that breakfast is the most important meal of the day. Eating meals low in fat and high in nutrients can help the body composition to maintain itself and provide the necessary building blocks for overall physical health. Eating a balanced diet will help you to have strong, shiny, healthy hair.

Hair begins under the skin in the dermal papilla— the root of the hair sac. The papilla contains cells that take in nutrition and amino acids, which are necessary for the hair to grow. The hair cells are produced in the matrix, which is the area above the papilla. The cells are pushed above the scalp while being produced in the matrix. At this point, the cells die and form into three layers: the medulla, cortex, and cuticle. The medulla is the innermost layer, which contains round cells. The cortex is the layer outside of the medulla, which contains dead cells, and a protein called keratin. The cuticle is the outermost layer that has seven overlapping layers of dead cells and keratin. After the initial growth process, it continues to grow through three phases: anagen (the active growth phase), catagen (the regressive phase), and telogen (the resting phase). During the anagen phase, the hair grows for many years and is vibrant and healthy. The hair is directly connected to a blood vessel, which gives the hair life. During the catagen phase, the hair stops growing, is pulling away from the papilla, and is no longer connected to the blood vessel. During the telogen phase, the hair is at rest and preparing to shed. This phase lasts for approximately two weeks. When a new hair begins to form, the cycle starts over again.

The elements of hair are two solids: sulfur and carbon, and three gases: nitrogen, hydrogen, and oxygen. Hair is also made up of about 90% protein.

Keeping Healthy Hair

When the outer layer of the hair follicle is damaged, the result could be hair loss. The damage happens because of the loss of keratin coupled with chemical processing that can cause the hair shaft to dry out because the protective "shingles" in the cuticle have been altered due to the chemical. The shingles on the cuticle tend to tangle with other pieces of hair causing breakage. If you chemically process your hair, you have to be careful in detangling to minimize breakage. Studies have shown that it is safer to detangle the hair with the fingers. In addition, natural hair can break as well if it is not properly moisturized.

Here are some tips to minimize breakage:

1. Use a satin or silk pillowcase to sleep on, or use a satin or silk bonnet to protect the hair.
2. Use a gentle natural soft bristle brush to style the hair.
3. Detangle the hair with the fingers as stated above.

Drink Water

Water plays a major part in the body's functioning. It is necessary to remove and flush out toxins from the body so that they do not settle within the hair. Many experts have stated to drink eight 8-ounce glasses of water per day for proper hydration.

Physical Fitness

Before starting ANY exercise program, always consult a physician. A physician can tailor an exercise program that would work for your body type and condition. The experts have stated that doing some moderate impact aerobic activity for 30-45 minutes four to five times a week is the recommended amount of exercise. Strength training exercises are important as well. It will help you to release specific hormones that make you look and feel younger. Body massages are helpful in stimulating blood flow and loosening up tight muscles to specifically targeted areas. A scalp massage can improve scalp condition and allow healthy hair growth because of blood flow stimulation to the scalp. A good thorough shampooing can make for a great scalp massage.

Exercise also allows you to release toxins and other impurities through your sweat glands further purifying your body in order to make the body strong. Also, Yoga has been known to aid people in maintaining a healthy weight. All of this plays a part in the health of your hair.

Many women of color do not do exercise because of the possibility of their hair becoming negatively affected by the exercise. Going to the beauty parlor and paying, in many cases, very expensive costs to get the hair done is often a deterrent from exercise because of the time and money spent on the hair appointment. I have heard many women say they are not going to do anything that would encourage them to sweat and, subsequently, "sweat out" their hair style. Even when some women go on vacation they find themselves not enjoying the water at the beach or engaging in too many activities that will encourage sweating. However, the women who get their hair braided or cornrowed before going on vacation will participate in water activities because they are not afraid of their hair becoming negatively affected by the activity.

Rest and Relaxation

Finally, your body needs daily rest in order to replenish and revitalize itself for the next day. Most people need six to eight hours of sleep every night in order to prevent fatigue and to allow the body to be able to function daily.

The Soul Aspect – Your Spiritual Health

God is our ultimate source of spiritual wellness. Therefore, getting in line with God is critical. The hair was a very important element back in biblical times. Many of the people during that time let their hair grow to great lengths. It was a symbol of strength for Samson who was reared under a specific Nazarite vow in which he was never to cut his hair or he would lose his incredible strength. In the story, God was true to his word and Samson did indeed lose his strength when, his love interest, Delilah cut off his hair so she could get money promised to her by the Philistines.

The lesson in this story is simple and it is two-fold. 1. God is true to his word and 2. There is an enormous amount of strength in our hair. When we do not properly care for the hair, the hair will most likely weaken and break.

Our conversations with God through prayer can help us to release the burdens that the world places on us each day. When we allow things like worry and fear to interfere with our daily living, it throws us out of balance causing an interruption in our conversations with God. He said that we should cast all of our worries (and stress) on him. The benefits of giving your stress to God outweigh you holding onto stress because stress can lead to hair loss. Meditating on scripture references like those at the end of this chapter can help with giving God your worry and stress.

In addition to prayer, the maintenance of spiritual wellness can be achieved through meditation. It is helpful in connecting the mind and body together with the soul. It can put you in a calm state and enhance you spiritually. Try this through Yoga.

After all is said and done, we can achieve healthier hair by using some basic techniques. Some things that you can do to maintain a healthy head of hair are wind down by listening to calming music, and concentrate on positive things. Release your daily stress through deep breathing, eat properly, exercise, drink water, get plenty of rest, connect yourself with God through prayer and bible study, love yourself as well as others, meditate and read inspirational passages, make good choices so that you have a clear conscience, be forgiving, laugh a lot, and share your testimony and faith with others. Although staying positive in a negative world can be difficult, you must try to in order to maintain not only the health of your hair but the health of your life—your mind, body, and soul. In order to function well, the mind, body, and soul need to be working together in unity. Remember, balance is crucial!

Scriptures for meditation

Be strong and of good courage, do not fear nor be afraid of them; for the LORD your God, He is the One who goes with you. He will not leave you nor forsake you." Deuteronomy 31:6

The LORD is my light and my salvation; whom shall I fear? The LORD is the strength of my life; of whom shall I be afraid? Psalm 27:1

In God I have put my trust; I will not be afraid. What can man do to me? Psalm 56:11

Chapter 4

Hair Loss Issues:
The Complications of Alopecia

Alopecia is an autoimmune disease that causes the immune system to attack and destroy the hair follicles and, subsequently, this causes a person to be the victim of hair loss. There are three forms of Alopecia: Alopecia Areata (mild patchy hair loss on the scalp), Alopecia Totalis (loss of all scalp hair), and Alopecia Universalis (loss of scalp and all body hair including eyelashes, eyebrows, and nose hair). Approximately four million Americans both male and female from many ethnic backgrounds suffer Alopecia Areata.

The disease can occur in people who have family members who suffer from other autoimmune diseases like Thyroid Disease, Type 1 Diabetes, Lupus, Psoriasis, or Rheumatoid Arthritis. Alopecia is not a contagious disease. However, it has genetic implications. Many people with immediate family members who have the disease have an increased risk of contracting the disease as well.

Although Alopecia is not life threatening, the affects of it can be emotionally devastating. The disease is unpredictable because it can come and go. The hair that was lost may or may not grow back.

Currently, Alopecia has no cure. Temporary treatments such as particular steroids and topical ointments exist that are available to possibly aid in helping the hair grow back, but there are no guarantees. Other ways to help to ease the discomforts of the disease are to use sunscreens, wigs, scarves, and hats when the hair on top of the head is missing. When other hair is affected like eyelashes, eyebrows, and nostril hair, experts say that you should wear sunglasses and use an antibiotic ointment in the nostrils to protect the nose.

Research is occurring in order to find a cure for the disease. If you are interested in finding out more information about Alopecia or hair loss in general, the website addresses are:

- The National Alopecia Areata Foundation www. naaf.org

- Help 4 Alopecia www.help4alopecia.com

- Traction Alopecia www.traction-alopecia.com

Chapter 5

The Hair Care Industry

The hair care industry is a $15 billion dollar industry. With companies like Dudley Products, Bronner Brothers, JM Products, Luster Products, and Soft Sheen-Carson, these companies will continue to be successful due to the types of products that they sell to African American's for the enhancement of African American hair. Products like relaxers, shampoo, conditioner, hairdressing, mousse, gel, leave-in conditioner, permanent hair color, styling and other finishing agents are items that African American women (and men) buy in abundance. Every product and company selling the product has their own unique marketing pitch to the public, which keeps them successful. What I find difficult and sometimes confusing is choosing the right product for my hair type, and the product that will suit my needs. Choosing carefully by reading the label on the product is important. Modern-day beauty salons and barbershops usually have many products on hand that they use on their clients' hair and sell to their clients. Beauticians and Barbers can be helpful in assisting you with purchasing the right product for your hair type.

Beauty Salons/Barber Shops

Many of us have seen the recent releases of the movies "Beauty Shop" starring Queen Latifah and the previous "Barber Shop" hits starring Ice Cube and Cedric the Entertainer. Beauty parlors and barbershops both provide great entertainment, unlimited conversation, and an open door policy allowing all to enter and leave as they please including those soliciting business for an item or items they are selling. We have all seen the salesmen/women coming in to sell women's handbags, hats, various types of clothing, CD's, food, etc. Many things that you can imagine are available for purchase through a number of beauty salons or barbershops. Some salons even have beauty supply stores within the salon. All of these scenarios do add a certain amount of flavor to the beauty salon/barbershop culture.

Although many modern-day salons can be a place of one-stop shopping, some of these situations can also be a recipe for disaster when there are too many shopping establishments within the salon. For example, I went to a salon that offered a photography studio, a hat/handbag store, a game room, and a beauty supply store all in one location. This set up was great for one-stop shopping but not so great because of loitering. In many cases, people would come to this shop and just stand around and converse all day, play pool, etc. What is bad in this situation is the loiterer may not have a scheduled appointment or any intention of being a walk-in customer, which could have a negative impact on a beautician or barbers scheduled appointments. Some people went there for the entertainment that the salon provides and to hang out which can be a distraction to the beautician. For example, if the beautician had a customer in the chair getting their hair done, sometimes the process would take longer than it should due to the distraction of the loiterer.

The loiterer would sometimes engage in conversation with the beauticians or barbers as they were serving customers. Ironically, there was a "no loitering" sign on the wall at this establishment. I also noticed in this salon that there was a sign on the wall that stipulated "no foul language," but customers AND OPERATORS alike would use foul language anyway.

Beauty parlors and barbershops are places where people meet and relationships form, receive therapy (for the mind), and listen to and participate in interesting conversation. They are usually well attended on the busiest days that are Thursday, Friday, and Saturday. Women go to get the latest and greatest hairstyle for purposes of going out with friends, dating, professional situations, self-pleasure, etc. Men go to get that "fresh" cut for the some of the same reasons as women.

Here is a note of caution, be prepared to spend quite a bit of time in a salon because they can be crowded and some stylists overbook so you wind up waiting, at times, after you scheduled an appointment. Sometimes this can happen regularly causing the customer to expect to wait for unreasonable amounts of time. In addition, some distractions, like lunch breaks, can get in the way of a scheduled appointment. At times, the beautician can put you on hold while eating lunch because she overbooked her schedule causing everyone's appointment to be bumped into the next appointment time and so on. Beauticians tend to overbook in case some of their clients do not show up. Many people tend to put up with this out of desperation because of being in dire need of getting their hair styled or touched up in order to keep evening plans, like going out on a date, a special meeting, etc. I believe there are only a handful of people who will actually get up and leave a salon if their wait time is significantly past their initial appointment time.

One of my friends has her hair done in a very quick and easy style that only takes about 30-45 minutes from start to finish and she is in and out of the salon. She has scheduled appointments at many salons who have told her that they are timely, and she has discovered during her second visit that they are not as timely as they stated. When she finds this out, she leaves to search for a salon that can accommodate her. She has done this on more than one occasion.

From my own experiences, some of the negative experiences that I have encountered at beauty salons are...

1. Beauticians not keeping the scheduled appointment time—if we have an appointment for 10:00 A.M. the appointment should not be more than 15-20 minutes past the initial appointment time.

2. Customer arriving at the salon for his or her scheduled appointment and the beautician is late because she went to get her nails done, her hair braided, has issues with her children, etc.

3. Spending unreasonable times in the salon--sometimes, there are so many people booked for one appointment time that it causes customers to stay for up to six hours.

4. Beauticians continuing to chemically process damaged hair instead of informing the customer that the hair should not be processed at that time.

5. There is too much foul language, gossip, and loitering in some establishments.

6. When the beauty salon and barbershop are all in one and they become a pick-up joint, which could make for an uncomfortable situation for a customer.

7. Some places allow unlicensed beauticians to provide services to customers for which a license is needed, i.e. in the use of a chemical.

8. Sometimes customers do not get the exact style that he or she wanted. For example, giving the client an actual "hair cut" when all they asked the beautician to do was trim the ends. In addition, some beauticians give you the hairstyle that they want as opposed to the style that the customer asked for without explanation.

9. The establishment is unclean. This refers to garbage on the floor to be swept up by the custodian/receptionist such as water bottles and hair pomade jars.

10. Parking can be challenging to obtain if the shop is located in a downtown urban area.

In relation to point number four above, Lonnice Brittenum Bonner, author of *"Good Hair"* had a problem with a beautician who did not take the time to analyze her hair prior to chemically processing it and she stated that many of us rely on beauticians because they are the "professionals." Some beauticians do not provide the professionalism and general expertise that they should, subsequently causing clients to need a "magician" to fix the problems caused by unprofessional beauticians.

What might make salon visits more pleasurable is if beauticians try to foresee any possible service problems as it pertains to each customer. For example, in the case of overbooking, perhaps beauticians or the shop receptionist could confirm the customer's appointment the day before to make sure that they will keep the appointment before scheduling additional people at the last minute in one appointment time. I understand that their income is contingent upon the customer keeping their appointment, but effective communication is critical in solving the overbooking problems.

Some of the positive situations that I have encountered are...

1. The beautician that gives a warm-friendly greeting when customers arrive instead of a cold stare at customers

2. The beautician that stays within 15-20 minutes of the actual appointment time even if she is running behind schedule

3. The beautician who actually does warn the customer if their hair is too damaged to be

chemically processed the way they want at that time

4. The beautician who does the customer's hair the way the customer wants like clip the customer's ends instead of cutting the hair

5. The salon that is an environment free from gossip, foul language, and loitering by customers without an appointment

6. The salon that provides added incentives for customers, i.e. discounts for recommending other customers, refreshments, etc.

7. The beautician who explains what she is doing to the customer's hair before she does it

8. The salon that allows you to purchase beauty supplies at a reasonable cost

9. The salon that is a CLEAN environment free from debris on the floor

10. The salon that is a PROFESSIONAL establishment, making it one in which the customers are treated with respect and will be pampered in the process

Communication is a very important tool in everyday operations. In the textbook "Salon Fundamentals," the author details several points to aid in effective communication between beauticians and customers. These points are: provide a pleasant greeting, use tact, express your ideas clearly, define the purpose of your communication, know the importance of your ideas, be aware of your environment, watch your overtones, consult with others when necessary, and be a good listener. These key points can aid in less misunderstandings between the beautician and customer. It is also stated in the textbook that beauticians should avoid discussing the following topics: religion, politics, personal problems, other client's behavior, staff or competitor's workmanship, and information told to the beautician in confidence. Many times, I have heard these topics being discussed in the salon, which I found to be quite unprofessional. Also, as stated in the textbook, some of the keys to a successful beautician/client relationship are...

1. Provide an explanation to the client of what the finished look will be;

2. Teach the client how to maintain their style at home;

3. Suggest that the client makes gradual instead of dramatic changes;

4. Give the client the option to reschedule if the beautician will be out on the day of their scheduled appointment instead of scheduling them with a fellow beautician.

I had an experience at a marvelous salon about 10 years ago named *"The Blueprint"* which was located in Somerset, New Jersey. The owner of the shop, Pam, was the only beautician who worked in the establishment—drama-free! I was impressed by her communication with customers about how their hair would handle different processes. She never overbooked clients and spaced out each appointment perfectly. She did not schedule appointments during her lunch hour or any other time that she would not be at the shop. She also made confirmation calls to her customers to make sure that the customer would keep the appointment. Her business was so organized that she had a waiting list of clients trying to get an appointment with her. Her waiting area was very comfortable with soft chairs, recent magazines, and soft music playing in the background. I liked the fact that her shop was clean, not overrun with customers, and there was no ridiculous gossip. She was extremely professional, and I would have stayed with her if she did locks. Unfortunately, according to my experience, this type of salon is the exception instead of the rule.

Another salon named *All About Gloria's* located in Somerset, New Jersey, is a great salon. First, appearance is everything to me so I was very impressed by the shop's cleanliness. I never saw hair on the floor or other debris. Items are swept up immediately. This is a quaint and lovely shop with a warm atmosphere. The furniture is not worn out, and everything has a professional edge to it, which I found to be delightful. The shop owner, Ms. Gloria, treats her customers with respect and does not overcharge for anything. This shop is not overrun with "stuff" and everything is in place. She has the ability to connect with her customers and provides them with high-level service. My daughter was a customer at this shop.

Both *The Blueprint* and *All About Gloria's* are symbolic of shops in the past—similar to the type of shop where my grandmother used to work in Newark, New Jersey—one that was classy and peaceful and that showed its customers respect in return for their business.

Prior to taking my daughter to *All About Gloria's*, I took her to a shop that had a nice appearance, but wound up being a disappointment because it was too costly and there were different hair dressers doing my daughter's hair which contributed to her having some major chemical damage to her hair. One day, my daughter had an appointment to get a touch up on her relaxer. We were informed that there was no hot water to rinse her hair, but if my daughter did not have a problem with lukewarm to cool water then they could still do her hair. Since she was at the point of needing her touch up and did not have a problem with lukewarm to cool water, we decided to get the touch up. Later, my daughter told me the water was cold not lukewarm. A few days later, I discovered she had major breakage. When she went back for a protein treatment, the beautician/shop owner who was supposed to do her hair stated that she did not know what my daughter was doing wrong with her hair but she had a large amount of breakage. By doing some researching and speaking with professionals, I found out that a chemical should never be washed out with cool water because it does not get the hair's Ph balance back in order. Putting the hair back in proper Ph balance means the relaxer's continual straightening power is turned off and the hair goes back into proper order. If the chemical is still active, then the hair becomes over processed leading to breakage. This was a nightmare because she had breakage on one side of her head so bad, it broke out down to the scalp also causing her hair to thin out terribly. She has recovered from that incident. She will <u>never</u> go to that shop again.

In the past, there was a time when the African American hair salon had a monopoly on providing services to African American customers. Now it seems that Hispanic salons are on the rise and serving not only the Hispanic community but the African American community. These shops are doing client's hair at prices, which are lower than their African American counterparts. From an economic standpoint, African American shops need to look at ways of providing service that is more competitive to the African American clientele in order to keep those clients. Shamboosie, author of "Beautiful Black Hair," has provided guidance to beauticians on professionalism.

According to Shamboosie, a true professional beautician should be able to tell you what you currently have in your hair and know the following:

1. If you have on a wig or a weave

2. If your relaxer is lye or no lye

3. If you retouched your own relaxer

4. If your hair is severely damaged

5. If you have been using cheap hair products

6. If you are using the wrong oils in your hair and using them the wrong way

7. If your hair can grow full, long, and healthy

8. If you have been given a bad hair cut

Also, he stated that people should use products in the same brand name family because they are designed to work together. Be careful to watch out for unlicensed beauticians applying chemicals to clients' hair. In addition, watch out for licensed beauticians who do not know how to apply chemicals properly to clients' hair.

In addition, Shamboosie also suggests when you are selecting the right salon you must do the following:

1. Ask for referrals from other people.

2. Ask a hairstylist for recommendations.

3. Visit different salons in the area.

4. Look for stylists who have many clients and observe their work.

If you are going to use chemicals in your hair, make sure that a true professional applies them because all chemicals can be damaging even if they are boxed and state that they are mild and can be applied by anyone. It takes about two years to replace hair damaged by no-lye relaxers. It is also suggested that if applying chemicals, that the hair not be bone straight. It will be much easier to style the hair if it still has a little of the natural curl in it.

Experts say that a conditioning lye relaxer is better than a no-lye relaxer because it leaves the hair soft and allows moisture to penetrate the hair shaft while relaxing. No-lye relaxers cause calcium build up, which locks the cuticle not allowing moisture into the hair shaft. This can lead to extreme dryness and, ultimately, breakage.

Essentially, the choice is yours whether you decide to go to a salon or not. Even though certain customers have negative experiences at some salons, this is not intended to say that these negative situations occur more often than not. You can judge for yourself those establishments that are treating their customers with the respect that they deserve. You can also judge for yourself whether your beautician is a "true professional" and knows what he or she is doing. Implementing things like open dialogue will aid in changes that can be made to improve particular establishments. I intended to provide this information so that negative situations become fewer and fewer and, hopefully, experiences that are more positive will occur at the beauty salon and barbershop that you decide to become a customer.

Antoinette Shar'ron Johnson

The Korean and Black Connection

According to an article written by Adrienne P. Samuels in the May 2008 edition of Ebony Magazine, in the 1970's and 1980's, 2nd generation Koreans began to open stores that sold wigs in the urban communities. That ambition allowed them to thirst for more which made them progress into the selling of black hair care products. Those stores gained popularity as women of African descent became more and more creative with their hairstyles and as supply and demand for extension hair and other products became popular. In order to achieve success, the stores were concentrated in urban areas. What is interesting about this scenario is that although African American people make up only 13% of the United States population, they make up 30% of the people who purchase products from these stores and other stores.

In the 1980's, the black hair care market initially started with African American-owned manufacturers. A number of those companies sold to white-owned companies. Currently, Korean distributors control a huge portion of the black hair care market and are the owners of over 9,000 stores to date.

The black hair care market has room for more African American ownership of distribution companies, manufacturing companies, and retail stores. In Somerset, New Jersey, Pro Beauty Supply is an African American-owned shop that has been in business for over 20 years. It is refreshing to know that African American ownership still exists and is able to keep up with the competition of other stores that sell black hair care products. This gives hope to those African American people who are considering becoming entrepreneurs of beauty supply stores. The African American community has to keep the beauty supply businesses open so they do not feel pressed to sell their businesses because of the financial reasons.

What about Hair Shows?

They are extravagant, extraordinary, fresh, vibrant, and quirky. The black hair show has been around for a little over 60 years and is still going strong! Hair shows were born around the year 1947 and was the brainchild of Bronner Brothers owners, Dr. Nathaniel H. Bronner, Sr. and Arthur E. Bronner, Sr. It started out at the Butler Street YMCA in Atlanta, Georgia, as a trade show with approximately 300 people in attendance. Since its inception, hair shows have grown in attendance to hundreds of thousands of people. The Bronner Bros. Empire has been passed onto Mr. Bernard Bronner who currently hails as CEO of the company.

Since the hair show's inception, they have taken on an edginess that is similar to fashion shows. Essentially, the hair show is a fashion show for hair fully equipped with a runway and a master or mistress of ceremonies. They usually take place over a three- to four-day period allowing various events to take place. These events include an exhibit hall for vendors, the hair show, a fashion show, workshops, boot camp for stylists, seminars, classes, nail and make-up sessions, and competitions for cosmetologists. The exhibitors could represent many industries such as media, hair care, wholesale, jewelry, fashion, fragrances, and cosmetics. These action-packed events can also include comedy or music concerts, various other forms of entertainment, and tours around town to see the historical landmarks. For the spiritual crowd, there may also be church service available.

The energy and excitement that occurs at hair shows is so high causing the guests to attend year after year. Hairstylists at these shows get to create some of the most innovative hairstyles with the assistance of the hair model.

Today, hair shows have become mega expos filled with vendors from across the country and have also taken on an international flair. Countries such as Denmark, Burkina Faso, and South Africa have joined the cause allowing for the dynamic styling of black hair to infiltrate internationally. In addition to the Bronner Bros. Hair Show in Atlanta, GA, some of the current well-known shows today include Rhythm & Style in Rockford, IL, and Hair Wars one of the largest hair shows in the country taking place in the fashion capital of the country, Detroit, MI.

Hair shows have taken on notoriety in the entertainment industry. The movie entitled, "Hair Show" starring *Mo'nique* and *Kellita Smith* was created to depict the dynamics of the hair show and was quite realistic.

In bringing the company into the 21st century and keeping with new technology, the Bronner Bros. Company has added to the company's resume online shows that highlight online classes, which are great learning opportunities for today's beauticians and barbers.

Chapter 6

The People Perspective

Your Family and Friends

What do you do when your family and friends do not understand the choice that you decided to make concerning your hair? With so many opinions, it can get confusing if you do not focus on what the bottom line, which is – keeping more hair on your head than on the floor, in the comb, or brush. Lonnice Brittenum Bonner, author of *"Good Hair,"* stated that she had some positive and negative comments from family members when she decided to go natural. She stated that when she went cold turkey and cut off all of her hair, her husband loved the short natural style and he particularly loved running his fingers through it, but some of her relatives were not too pleased with her choosing the natural style. It seems that people tend to believe they have been betrayed in some way if a person decides to go natural. Maybe people feel uncomfortable because of the negative experiences concerning "nappy hair" that they have dealt with throughout their lives.

When individuals choose a natural style, some people will not like it and some people will think your natural style is "cool." In many cases, people say negative things because they are uncomfortable with it, and they do not have a full understanding of what the natural style truly represents to you. The bottom line is YOU have to be happy.

Corporate America:
The J-O-B and Job Discrimination

I have noticed over time that there has been a change in the climate concerning women in the corporate arena and the desire to wear natural hairstyles. Johnson & Johnson (J&J) is a great example of a corporation allowing their employees to express their ethnic diversity. In fact, they promote and support it. When I visited J&J for a community service program one evening, I was very impressed to see that African American women were not only wearing short naturals but they were wearing braids and even locks! Here is a brief history of African American hairstyle trends and how they were received by corporate America:

In the 1960's and 1970's
The afro was popular.

In the late 1970's
The cornrow started receiving popularity largely due to, actress Bo Derek who wore them in the movie "10."

In the 1980's
Braids were not well received in all corporate arenas.

In the 1990's
Braids/Cornrows started to become accepted in Corporate America.

In the 2000's
Locking and other natural styles are accepted by Corporate America.

Largely due to the Civil Rights Act of 1964, the corporate structure is not allowed to dictate that employees must wear a certain hairstyle as long as the hair is neat, clean, well groomed, and meets length requirements if there are any. Ultimately, many people have filed lawsuits against corporations because some corporations have overstepped their bounds by telling employees, especially African Americans, how they are allowed to wear their hair. In the corporate arena, it has always been a struggle for African American women to go natural because they want to stick with what is "comfortable" and non-confrontational in their place of employment. African Americans are more likely to be told to conform to another's style if their current style appears to be confrontational. Even if people do not agree with the "policy" it takes a strong, confident woman to stand up to the authorities and make, in fact, what is deemed to be a political statement.

Some of the lawsuits occurred because corporations violated the employee's rights under Title VII of the Civil Rights Act of 1964. In fact, according to the Equal Employment Opportunity Commission (EEOC), Title VII of the Civil Rights Act of 1964 says, "Discrimination on the basis of an immutable characteristic associated with race, such as skin color, hair texture, or certain facial features violates Title VII."

In 2003, a college-educated African American man was employed at a corporation in Atlanta, Georgia that employed 90% African Americans. His African American supervisor asked him if he would consider cutting his locks in order to look "more professional" and "fit in" with the company atmosphere. He did not agree to it, and his supervisor dropped the subject. Then, he was told (after some time went by) to cut the locks because "upper management" wanted them to be cut. The policy stated that men must have their hair above the collar line, and nothing indicated the "type" of hairstyle that men were or were not allowed to wear. This case was presented before the EEOC for investigation. At this time, there is no further information about the case. In this case, it appears that the supervisor was possibly afraid that his job would be in jeopardy if he did not get the employee to comply with the company's demands.

As I was walking through the airport one day, a Flight Attendant walked past me, and I noticed her hair was locked. Not only was she wearing locked hair, but also it was short and colored blond. Flight Attendants are also cutting their hair to short natural styles and they are adding color to their short natural styles.

What we should realize is that a company policy cannot be used to control or bully an employee into doing something (in this case, to their hair) that is more "comfortable" or "acceptable" to the upper level management. As was stated earlier, as long as the hair is neat, well groomed, clean, and meets the length requirements, a style cannot be chosen for the individual that will be wearing the style. That means you can wear your hair in the short afro, two-strand twists, braids, cornrows, locks, etc. as long as you meet the basic standards. In my review of company policies, I found that one in particular stated that an employee had to maintain a "neat, clean, well-groomed personal appearance in order to make an appropriate impression upon the company, the peers, and the public" and did not specifically refer to an employees hair. The policy also states that employees have the right to work in an environment free from objectionable and disrespectful conduct, discriminatory harassment, ridicule, etc. Anyone who feels they have been subjected to this negativity can go to his or her supervisor or next person in charge of their department to report it. If no positive results are seen, then the employee may decide to seek outside legal counsel and, ultimately, the EEOC.

On the flipside, I have discovered in my travels that if you go to an interview with a hairstyle that is viewed upon as "militant" such as locks or a braided style that may prevent you from getting the job. Unfortunately, discrimination still exists to a certain degree. I decided to lock my hair after I worked at my current job for seven years. When I started working at my current place of employment, my mindset was different and, I was not thinking about locking at that time.

Your Co-workers

In reference to my locked hair, I ran into an Italian-American person where I work. He said to me in utter disgust, "Why did you do that to your hair?" My first response was, "Do what?" I then replied to him that I decided to work with my natural hair, which was better for me. He proceeded to shake his head as though I have betrayed, threatened, or offended HIM in some way. He also was misinformed and called my locked style "cornrows." I was unable to respond to his ignorance with more information as his co-worker distracted me with a non-related issue.

In addition, I will never forget the time that another person of African descent saw my locks for the first time. She approached me with a look on her face as though I had committed a crime. When people of African descent give negative stares, it shows that we have not come as far as we should have in supporting each other in different things especially those things that take a considerable amount of strength and courage to do. People have uncomfortable feelings that they are not dealing with concerning natural hair, and that is the reason why they react the way that they do. I was very disappointed by the negative look this person gave me especially because it came from a person of African descent.

Lastly, a Russian woman at my place of employment made a negative comment. To paraphrase, she asked me if I could take my hair out [of its locked state] because, according to her, I could be much "more beautiful" if I do different things to my hair. She made it a point to inform me, that she would do many different things to her hair when she was younger, i.e. color it, cut it, etc. Also, she asked if I could wash my hair. I informed her that I have done all of the things that I wanted to do to my hair, and I am very pleased with it as it is currently. I also explained to her that I shampoo and condition my hair as everyone else does. I like when people ask questions so that I can dispel any myths, untruths, and ignorance concerning locked hair. The questions she posed were in a condescending way and that is what made it feel more like an interrogation rather than just inquiring conversation. The instance with the Russian person and the Italian-American person are clearly, what I will call cases of cross-cultural ignorance, which is what I define as a condition of being uneducated, unaware, or uninformed about another's culture, and harboring untrue beliefs about that culture. Cross-cultural ignorance has the potential to lead to discrimination. In today's world, it is vital to understand that individuals from other ethnic groups or cultures have ceremonies, rituals, rules, and values that differ from one's own and that is fine.

On a positive note, the Russian woman also gave me a compliment about my locked hair. One day I came in with my hair pulled back in a bun. She actually said to me "I like your hair like that." What that meant was she was more comfortable with my hair pulled back into a bun as opposed to flowing down past my shoulders. Maybe it was less threatening to her in the "bun" style.

People who wear their hair natural experience those types of negative comments from day to day. Listening to these comments puts some things into perspective. We must understand the root of the comments and that most comments are in relation to ignorance. When we do not understand something about another culture and do not engage in dialogue about that which we do not understand, that can lead to insensitive comments, disrespect and, ultimately, hard feelings. What I have also found is if someone does not like your hair, then he or she may not say anything at all about it and that is fine. That is probably the best way to handle that situation. I have also received some very positive statements about how nice my hair is. Believe me it always helps to hear positive things! It provides balance.

Chapter 7

Women's and Men's Perspective on Hair Processes Survey

I conducted a random survey to get a sense of what women have gone through and are going through pertaining to the various hair processes they may have tried. Also, I wanted to get a sense of what men felt about the choices that the women in their lives make concerning their hair. To capture the information, I developed a web-based survey, which allowed women and men to answer the questions online anonymously. After the survey participant submitted the online form, the answers would transmit into a database without participant identifiers in order to maintain confidentiality. This process was successful and yielded over 80 responses. As you will see, some of the results are broken down into bar graphs for better visualization.

The Women....Statistics and General Comments

During the process, I surveyed women on the various types of styles: Braids and Cornrows, Chemical Processes (Relaxer and Curly Perm), Locks, other Natural styles (not including Locks and

Braided/Cornrowed styles), Pressed styles, Weaves and Wigs. The statistical portion of this survey was quite interesting.

The survey participants included 66 women of African descent that ranged in age from late teen to 75 years of age. The women's survey was very interesting and allowed me to confirm some common things that women go through. I found out women of color, in general, like a variety of styles. The majority of responses were from women who relaxed their hair and the lowest response came from a woman who prefers to wear a weave. Some women have more than one style that they are wearing, i.e. relaxer and braids. Since the survey was not designed to capture information on a person who may be wearing multiple styles, participants were asked to choose the style that they wear most often to ensure one survey per person has been completed.

Some of the major problems that I found out were not having their hair done the way that they wanted by their beautician, over processing hair causing breakage, use of permanent hair color causing dryness, brittleness of hair, dependency upon chemical processes, being burned on the scalp by the relaxer cream, and unlicensed beauticians operating and using chemicals on patrons. Because of these conditions, some of the women were in the process of converting from the relaxer to natural.

One woman stated that she cut all of her hair off by choice, let it grow back, and then put a relaxer back in it because, as she stated, "the natural did not complement her." However, even though she stated her hair was thicker and healthier when it was in its natural state, she still chose a chemical process for her hair. Another interesting comment came from a woman who stated that she chooses to relax her hair because of her "conservative career" and that a natural hairstyle is actually her preference but she adjusts because of her career. In addition to this woman's comment, another woman said she likes the "professional appearance achieved with relaxer and weaved styles."

Even though one woman prefers the natural hairstyle instead of the relaxer because her hair is thinner relaxed, she still relaxes her hair. Other reasons pertained to women feeling that their hair is more manageable in a relaxed state and one woman prefers the "long straight look."

Another woman stated that even though she wears the relaxed hairstyle, she prefers the hair weave because, for the most part, the weather does not affect the style.

BRAIDS AND CORNROWS

Regarding the participants for the braids and cornrows survey, the majority of the participants were born and raised in the USA. Half were married and the other half were single.

Based upon a scale of like, dislike, unsure, and no comment, all who participated on the braids/cornrows survey liked locks, relaxers, and other natural styles. Whereas, only half liked the weave and three-quarters liked wigs.

Although they were wearing their hair in a braided style, three-quarters of them preferred chemical process over natural styles, did not keep up with fad styles, and experienced hairline breakage. Half of them go to salons as opposed to having their hair done at a non-professional location, experienced hairline breakage and only half were satisfied with the length of time the style lasts. None of the women heard negative comments pertaining to their hairstyle. Most have worn braids from one to 10 years.

Some of the other comments pertained to professional locations being very expensive. It was also stated that synthetic hair caused thinning and breakage to some of their hair as opposed to human hair. Swimming has caused damage to one woman's hair due to the reaction between the chlorine and the braids.

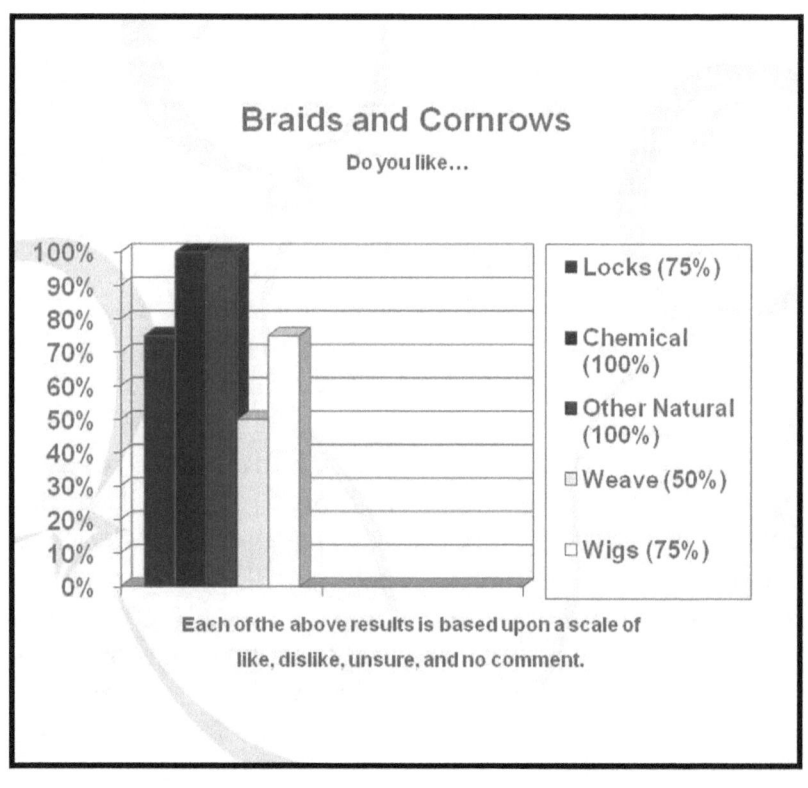

Braids and Cornrows
Do you like...

- Locks (75%)
- Chemical (100%)
- Other Natural (100%)
- Weave (50%)
- Wigs (75%)

Each of the above results is based upon a scale of like, dislike, unsure, and no comment.

CHEMICAL PROCESSES

The two main processes surveyed were the curly perm (i.e. Jheri Curl®) and relaxer. The majority of responses came from the women who preferred the relaxed style. Based upon a scale of like, dislike, unsure, and no comment, most liked the relaxed style, braids and cornrowed styles, and did not keep up with fads. Three-quarters liked the other natural styles, some liked hair weaves, less than half liked wigs, and a little more than half liked locks.

The survey results showed that the majority of women liked the relaxer over the curly perm. Concerning hair salons, over half actually go to a salon and over three-quarters are satisfied after going to a salon. Those women who were, in fact, satisfied with going to a salon stated they did not experience extreme breakage or baldness due to the use of chemicals. More than half did not experience other problems from the chemical. Even though more than half did not experience other problems, more than one-quarter did and that is too high of a number in my opinion. The women surveyed have worn their hair in a chemical process from less than one year to over 15 years.

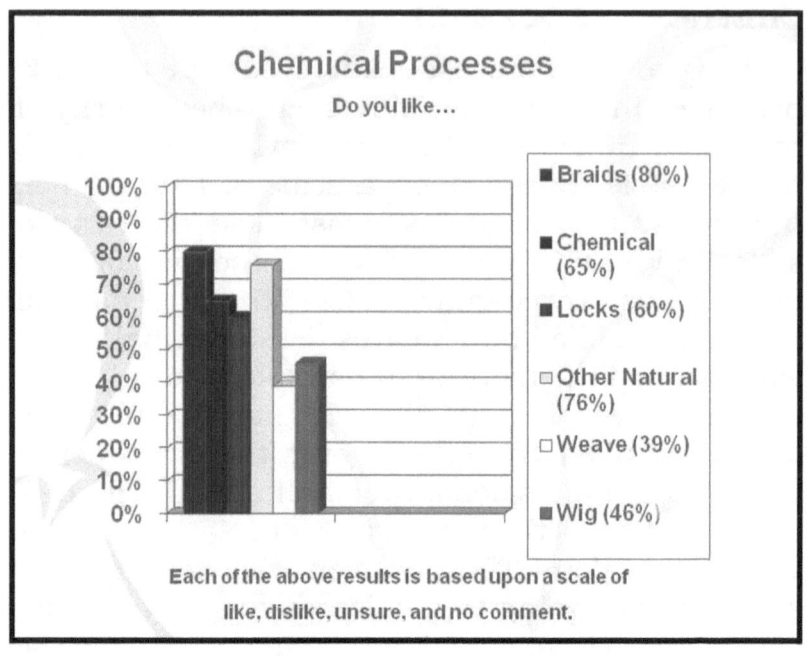

LOCKED STYLES

The locked hairstyle has started taking on a trend that has not been seen since braiding became popular. More and more women are wearing their hair locked than have for over 20 years ago. The women surveyed have worn their hair locked less than a year to up to 15 years. Some people think of this style as more of a radical style because it is viewed as being extreme.

It compares to the afro worn in the 60's in terms of its extremeness. Many of the women are choosing to lock because it preserves their hair from the damage that chemical processes can cause. They like locks because it is easy to care for, convenient, versatile, keeps the hair healthy, helps them to stay connected with their race, and they just like the naturalness of the style.

I found that 100% of the women surveyed who wear locks were married. The majority wore their hair locked for themselves as opposed to anyone else. In a comparison between the relaxer and the curly perm, based upon a scale of like, dislike, unsure, and no comment, three-quarters liked relaxers and disliked curly perms, which I thought was very interesting. All liked naturals and braids and half disliked weaves. Out of all of the styles, the locked population preferred the locked style the most. They were not too impressed with beauty salons over all. Three-quarters did not keep up with fads, were satisfied with the length of time their hair lasts and did not have any other twisting problems. Half did their own hair and re-twisted their hair every 6-8 weeks. None had breakage problems. Three-quarters did not experience negative comments about their hair from the work place. One woman thought that the weave should only be worn when necessary and not as a permanent form of style.

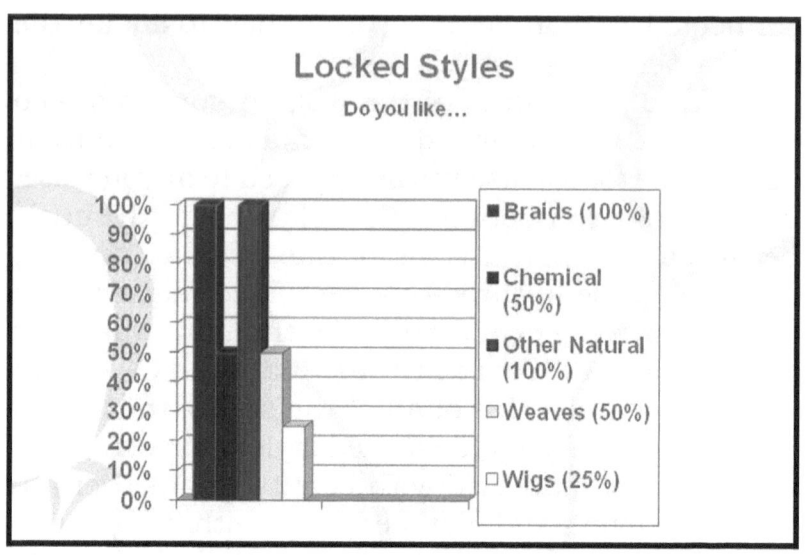

OTHER NATURAL STYLES

The natural styles section of the survey was based upon the short afro style or any other style not altered from its natural state by chemicals. This survey does not include the locks, braids, or cornrow styles since they have already been represented by the previous surveys.

I discovered in this survey that half of the participants were married. Based upon a scale of like, dislike, unsure, and no comment, more than half of the participants liked braids, weaves, wigs, and locks.

More than half of the participants felt satisfied after going to a salon, most did not change their style to keep up with fads, and most stated that they did not feel ashamed of their hair in its natural state. A disturbing fact that I discovered is half of the participants felt bad about their hair in its natural state and almost three-quarters have been caught up in the "good hair/bad hair syndrome." Many felt their natural hair is not difficult to handle and they have enough time to do their hair. Most are comfortable with their hair texture and more than half would not change anything about their hair. The women surveyed have been wearing their hair natural for less than 1 year to over 15 years.

Some of the women felt that their hair was too frizzy and would, therefore, like it to be less frizzy. One woman stated that she appreciates that her husband's does not dictate to her the style she should wear and she values his opinion. Concerning the good hair bad hair syndrome, unfortunately we still have barriers to overcome with this. One woman stated that she wished that she had her mom's hair because it was very long, down to the bottom of her back due to her American Indian heritage. Another woman stated that chemicals, no matter the strength, burn her scalp and she could not use them. She wears her hair natural because of that fact.

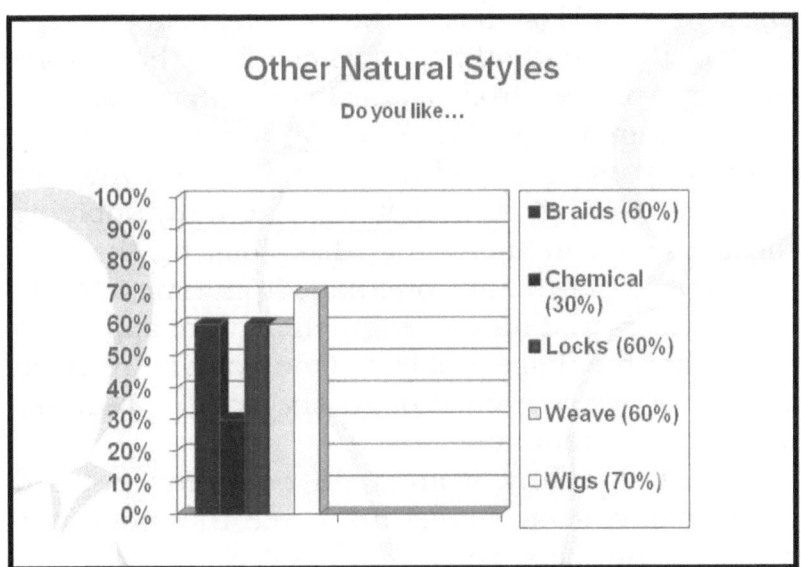

PRESSED STYLES

Although many women, due to the chemical processes, do not frequently wear pressed styles, I thought it would be interesting to find out if some of the women still have their hair pressed. It was my belief that some women still chose this type of style because the hair can easily go back to being natural without having to cut all of the hair off to get rid of chemically processed hair.

Of the women surveyed, more than half were born and raised in the USA and more than one-quarter were born and raised in the Caribbean. Also, more than one-quarter of the women were married, and more than half were widowed. Based upon a scale of like, dislike, unsure, and no comment, more than half liked relaxed styles. Half of the participants liked locks. All liked other natural styles and braids. More than half were satisfied with the length of time their hair lasted after going to a salon. Over half did not keep up with fad styles and did not have breakage. The style would last most of the women about 3 weeks. None of them had other problems. They have worn their hair pressed from 1 year to over 15 years.

One woman stated that her definition of pressing is actually using a conditioner and blow-drying her hair out to straighten it instead of actually applying the hot comb to the hair. Also, coloring the hair has caused her to have breakage from time to time. Moisturizers and hair strengtheners were applied to rectify her breakage problem. One woman preferred to wear a weave even though she presses because it's "low maintenance."

Although many women do not wear pressed styles today, it is interesting to see that some are still wearing the style!

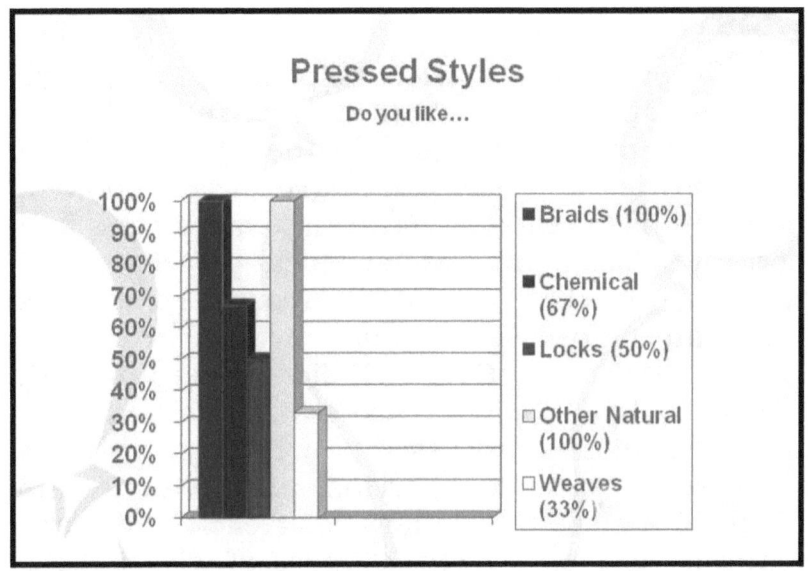

WEAVES

There was one woman who completed the survey for the hair weave. She stated that she likes the weave because it gives a professional appearance. She has had various problems from wearing it such as itchy scalp and her actual hair not remaining in place under the weave. She likes the fullness, length, and style that it gives as well as the protection it provides for her own hair. She did like the following styles, relaxers, natural, braids, and weaves. She was unsure how she felt about wigs and locked styles. She disliked the curly perm.

She prefers to wear the weave most of the time because she feels good after going to a professional salon and having it done. She has admitted to changing her hairstyle to keep up with fads. She has her hair done every eight weeks and is okay with that. She has been wearing her hair weaved for 11 to 15 years.

WIGS

Not very many women responded to the wig survey. Out of the women who did respond, over half were born and raised in the USA, over half were married and over one-quarter were widowed, over half liked relaxers, natural, weave, braids and cornrows, locks, preferred chemical processes, and were unsure about how they felt about the curl. Less than half of those women that wear wigs prefer their hair to be weaved. Over half did not keep up with fad styles, liked the wig because of its convenience, prefer chemically processed hair because it's more manageable, did not experience any breakage and all were satisfied with how long each wig lasts. Many liked the cost effectiveness of wigs. Some had problems with the wig not fitting properly. The women who participated in the survey have worn wigs for one year to over 15 years.

Regarding all the survey responses, many women have a desire to do what is best for their hair, but society sometimes makes it difficult to do so.

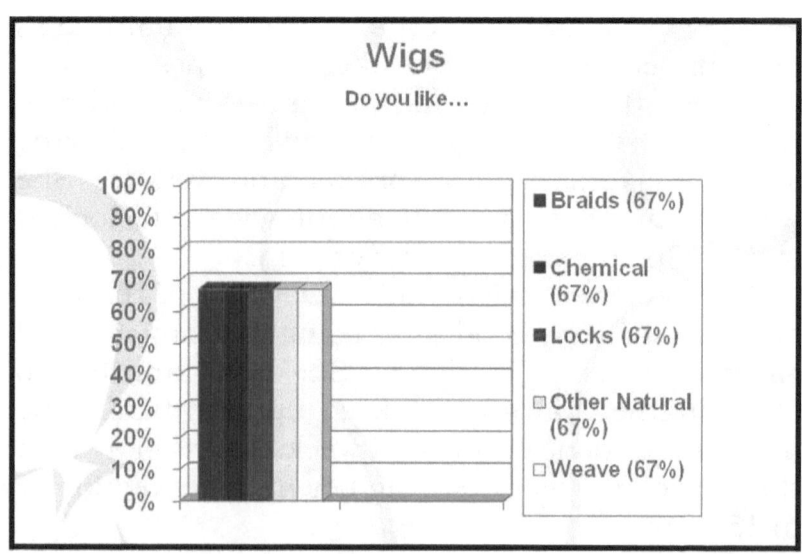

Overall, we have come a long way in our hairstyle choices. Good, bad, or indifferent, we all have choices that we can make when it comes to our hairstyles. I was not surprised to find out that the majority of the responses were for the chemically processed styles particularly the relaxer. It was interesting to find out that although some of the women had damaged hair due to the chemical process, many have given chemicals more than one chance. I was glad to find out that a large majority of the women who wore their hair in natural styles were not made to feel bad about their hair.

The Men...Statistics and General Comments

When I started to develop the web-based hair surveys, initially, I only had the women in mind. About half way through receiving the women's results, I realized that a very important source had not been tapped into...our men! I realized at that point that the men's opinions and responses were crucial and key to this book and women in general.

Believe it or not ladies, the male response is an important part of this whole process because we truly need to know how they feel about what we do and do not do to our hair. It is vital that we put aside our fears and find out what they truly think about the women in their lives. Many of us have been guilty of asking our boyfriends, husbands, etc. "So honey, how does my hair look?" The reality is, in some cases, we do not really want to know how they truly feel or we are hoping they will give us a positive response even if the style does not warrant a positive one. It is estimated that these men ranged in age from late teens to the mid 50's.

The following responses are based upon 15 men who were surveyed:

MORE THAN THREE-QUARTERS OF THE MEN....

--liked their wife or girlfriend's hair as it is currently styled.

MORE THAN HALF OF THE MEN...

--like natural styles instead of chemically processed styles.

--thought their wife/girlfriend spent too much time at the salon on any given appointment.

--said that it takes less than one hour for their wife/girlfriend to get ready if they are going out on a date, and they are okay with the time it takes their wife/girlfriend to get ready for a date.

LESS THAN HALF OF THE MEN...

--like long hair.

--like beauty salons.

--said that their wife/girlfriend pays too much money at the salon and the same amount of men said that they did not know how much is spent at the salon.

ABOUT ONE-QUARTER OF THE MEN...

--said that women spend 2-2 ½ hours at the salon.

--said that they spend 1-2 hours getting ready for a date.

--said that they are okay with the cost and more than one-quarter said that if the could choose a style for her it would be long.

--said if they could choose a style it would be short.

SOME OF THE MEN...

--like braids, short hair, afros, twists.

--said if they could choose a style it would be braids.

--said if they could choose a style for their wife or girlfriend it would be the afro, twist, or straight, and some were not sure.

--like what their wife or girlfriend likes.

Here are some additional interesting comments from the men's survey questions:

"Natural is preferred if your hair is "good" but if you hair is "bad" then you'll need a chemical."

"Well, I like her hair because it's easy. She can get dressed faster and doesn't have to use rollers."

"Hair needs to be done at all times whether you are going anywhere or not!"

"I liked the hair to be long and wild...no curls."

"I like beauty salons because they have a choice of different styles that you may want to see your lady in."

"Beauty salons are too time consuming."

"I love to play with her hair and run my fingers through it."

"If they [beauty salons] can find a way not to keep my wife half of the day I would love them more."

"I wish she would let it grow."

"She's never satisfied with her hair…it drives me crazy!"

"I'd rather her wear it natural because her hair texture is thicker than the "permed out" look."

"I think they [beauty salons] overcharge for what people want to have done."

Overall, the results and this entire process were very interesting to me. I was surprised to find out that more men prefer the natural styles (short afro, braids, locks, etc.) compared to the chemically processed styles and was happy to know that most men liked what their women do to their hair. I was not surprised to find out that many men are not happy with the amount of time women spend in beauty salons. On average, the men stated that the women are spending a little more than three hours in the salons on any given appointment. That amount of time is the norm. However, one man stated that his wife has spent as much as eight hours in a salon on a given appointment.

For additional survey results, please go to Appendices II and III.

Chapter 8

My Perspective, My Journey: Positive and Negative Experiences

For many years, I have been on the search for that perfect hairstyle—a style that is easy to work with yet one that would allow versatility with styling. I have been searching for a hairstyle that will allow for quick styling in order to get out of the house in a pinch. I realized that the reason for my experimenting with so many different hairstyles was because I was searching for something, but at first, I did not know what I was trying to find. It never occurred to me that I could achieve various styles with a hairstyle such as locking until I started looking for a style in the black hair care magazines. I also realized that relaxing my hair was damaging and that it took the body and definition out of my hair, but I was so focused on not dealing with my coarse textured hair so the straight style and damage outweighed having my hair natural and healthy. Because of my hair's coarseness, beauticians would process my hair until it was lifeless. The combination of heat products to my terribly fragile chemically processed hair was a recipe for disaster.

In my experience with locking, it seemed as though some people felt uncomfortable with my new style. They did not know what to call it. Some were calling it braids, others called it dreads, and others called it twists. In a twisted way, (no pun intended) some natural styles are viewed as being negative and some people believe that straightening their hair is what needs to be done and that is not necessarily the case. Straightening may work for some but not all. We should learn to be accepting and supportive of the choices that individuals make regardless of whether you agree or not agree. Truthfully, it is difficult for some to accept natural styles when they have been told that coarse hair texture is a curse or it is not beautiful. This hair journey is definitely a process.

During my lifetime, I have done it all: the pressing comb, Vigorol®, Carefree Curl®, Leisure Curl®, various relaxers, braids, short afro, etc. all the while searching for the best style for my hair. I figured I would try locking since that was the only thing left that I did not try. I believe my journey has taken this long so that I could truly appreciate who I am as an African American woman - a versatile woman. This journey has been a very spiritual one for me. I have had to learn to love myself for who I am, and it has not been easy. I will not say that it is wrong for someone to press out or relax their hair. I am not in a position to judge anyone nor do I want to. African American women are very creative, stylish, and innovative people. We have taken our hair to another level by creating some of the most interesting looking and fun hairstyles. What I am saying is we all have to find our path and be happy with whatever we decide.

When I decided to lock my hair, I was not trying to go against the status quo. I was trying to find an escape from the problems that I was experiencing with my hair. My main goals were to find a style that would help to preserve my hair, complemented me, and had a certain level of versatility.

There was a time when I believed that distinct African features were not a blessing. I had a problem with my wide nose, thick lips, and kinky hair, and there was a time when those features were not widely accepted in the real world. Actually, the real world is not as cruel a place as I thought. More and more of our traditions are being accepted. Once you assert yourself and show self-confidence, your beauty will come from the inside. If you feel beautiful, then you are beautiful. No longer will I be a slave to any particular process in order to live by someone else's definition of beauty. Everyone has a specific path to travel. It takes a lot of thought and research to make such a life-altering decision as locking because once the lock sets, it is permanent. The only way to remove locks is to cut them. Truthfully, speaking cutting my locks does not scare me. I am definitely a rebel. In my transition to locking, I just got tired of seeing my hair on the bathroom floor instead of on my head. I would never advise making this decision, or any other for that matter, without proper thought, research, and consultation with a beautician that specializes in natural hair care.

Concerning my daughter, I believe she has to make her own hair decisions and go through her own journey. Although I advise her of the good, bad, and ugly from my experiences, I want her to be her own individual and not an exact replica of me. Whatever choices she decides to make with her hair,

I will support her. Also, I will give her suggestions on safer and healthier hairstyle choices based upon my own experiences. In addition, I would never force her into locking her hair. I feel that everyone that has taken this journey into locking their hair has a real appreciation for what they have gone through to make the decision to lock. I discovered that locking is actually a type of spiritual awakening in which an epiphany occurs allowing you to see your previous experiences before making the decision to lock. One day she may be ready to make the transition. However, she will have to determine that for herself.

Sometimes we get so caught up in what the majority of the world is doing that we lose sight of what is right for us. As shown in history, there have been moments when African Americans have taken a bold stance against what the vast majority is doing and have dealt with negativity and ignorance.

Some African Americans think that by living in this society they cannot truly be who they are. Some people think that they cannot get a particular corporate position if they have natural hair. In some cases, you may not get that corporate position, but my belief is if you have been faithful to God then HE will not leave you nor forsake you. HE will supply all of your needs and you should believe that you will have the job that HE wants you to have. If you claim it, it is yours! Maybe the job that you set your eyes upon is not what God has in store for you. If you do not receive that job, look upon the situation as one that God is protecting you from for whatever reason and move on to the next prospect. You should understand that there is an underlying reason for everything.

You have to be happy with yourself and accept yourself in order for others to accept you. Truthfully, you may never "fit in" no matter how many changes you make to yourself. If you do not accept who you are, how do you expect someone else to accept you? You have to hold your head up high and feel good about who God has made you to be. People will respect you for the person you are if you display high self-esteem. My mother always said that people do not have to like you, but they do have to respect you. Demand respect and you will receive it! Confidence is the key. People have the right to do whatever they want with and to their hair. My suggestion is that you make sure that you are comfortable with your choice whatever that may be.

Also, understand that your hair is not always the real issue. Sometimes people try to gain control over. If you believe that your hair texture is the worst thing given to you, then you may change it. If you believe that your skin color is too dark, then you may lighten it. If you believe that your lips are too thick, then you may alter them. If you believe that your nose is too wide, then you may make it smaller. Many times when someone tries hard to change you from who you are those things that you view as weaknesses may actually be strengths. If you have some deep-seeded resentment about yourself, a hair weave will not make your resentment disappear. Re-examine yourself and then build upon your self-esteem.

After being told repeatedly of all of your so-called faults by your own people, sometimes you begin to believe them. A lot of the time, we commit black on black crime when we tell each other that we need to chemically process, add weave, or whatever.

The tearing down of someone's self-esteem is not only degrading but also disrespectful. We need to build each other up and support each other for the decisions that we make. Many people have a long way to go in that respect.

I reached a point in my life in which I understand what I want from a spiritual perspective, and I have made positive changes in my life for self-pleasure and enhancement. I am truly happy and satisfied with my decision to lock and have inner peace. My hair is symbolic of my inner strength and my true feelings about me. Before I made the change, my thoughts about myself were interconnected with others thought about me. Although it is important to me how my family and friends feel about me, the most important thing to me is how GOD views me, what GOD thinks about me, and what GOD has made me to be.

My level of self-esteem has grown tremendously because I made the change for me. In spite of my change, there is still a lot of ignorance out there. The best thing that I can do for a person who is displaying obvious ignorance towards me is to pray for them that they will learn not to be afraid of that which is different from them but to embrace differences and possibly learn something from what is different from them.

I feel such freedom with my hair because it is something that I did for self-preservation. I feel as though the shackles of slavery have come off, and I can truly be who God called me to be!

The Transition/Transformation - December 26, 2001

I went through a lot of blood, sweat, and tears prior to my transformation. As I already stated, I wore many other hairstyles before making the decision to lock. I have been through enough hair drama to last a lifetime. I appreciate those experiences because they have prepared me for where I am now in this hair journey. Women of African descent, put so much emphasis in the coif and need to be comfortable in their hair decisions. No way could I have locked my hair 20 years ago because I was not ready.

I have always been a chance taker and somewhat of a rebel. I will try many things at least once. I understood the societal risks involved with my transition to locks but that did not stop me from trying it. I have learned in my life not let fear of the unknown be a deterrent from the things that I would like to try. Being fearful would only cause me to not live to my full potential, and it goes against my faith and trust in God. However, I would not suggest anyone taking risks that are life threatening, but taking a risk on something that has the potential of changing your life positively should be taken.

When I was investigating what to do next, after reading hair magazines that showed how beautiful women looked with locked hair styles, I spoke with my friend Eloise "Dee Dee" Jacobs who had already locked her hair and gave me that boost to try it. That is when I realized that I should try locking. What did I have to lose?

Locking my hair has been a freeing experience. I can drive in my car and not worry about my hair messing up when the windows are down. Contrary to my days before locking, I can wake up, shower, and go without fussing too much over my hair.

Until now, I did not realize that I could feel confident with my hair in its natural state. I always thought my hair was too coarse or nappy to look right in a natural style. One thing that I needed to have was versatility. I needed a natural style that would allow me to wear a ponytail, bun, etc. There is a lot of versatility with this hairstyle.

Stages of Locking

In reference to my experience, there are a few steps to consider in the locking process. I first allowed my relaxed hair to grow out and would trim a little off each time I washed and conditioned my hair. Once all of the relaxer was out, I went to a professional beautician to begin the locking process.

I must admit that I was both excited and nervous at the same time about the process. Even though I had my hair cut short before, I did not know what to expect with this new style. I hoped it would look nice and suit my face. Truly, I saw my hair in a different light, and I liked it from the very beginning.

On the day that changed my life, December 26, 2001, the beautician twisted my hair with a special locking cream, used a metal clip to hold my individual twists in place, and then I sat under the dryer to allow my hair to set. After I came out from under the dryer, she removed the clips, sprayed my hair with a little oil and off I went. It was pain free!

For those of you contemplating locking your hair, the following are the formal stages of locking: Phase 1: The Pre-lock or Baby Stage. This is the beginning stage where you have numerous small spirals all over the head. Phase 2: The Budding

Phase or Teen Stage—at this stage, the hair is still pre-locked and is starting to lengthen often having a mind of its own. Phase 3: The Shooting Phase or Adult Stage—this is the stage where the hair begins to interlock and starts to become dense. The hair remains in this stage for the longest time. Phase 4: Contracting Phase or Elder Stage—at this stage, the hair is completely locked and cannot be unraveled.

Myths

I wanted to touch on this subject because a few myths that are going around about locked hair need to be dispelled. Some people believe that locked hair is unclean and unwashed which is not true. I wash and condition my hair like everyone else.

Another myth to dispel is the fact that locks and dreadlocks are the same thing. Dreadlocks are a style worn mostly by Rastafarians (a religious sect) and can vary in size and shape and Locks are the cousin of the dreadlock, are the same size, and shape as seen in American and other cultures. In addition, contrary to what some believe, people who wear locks are not necessarily Rastafarian.

Is Locking Permanent?

As far as I know, after doing research, locking is a permanent process. Recently I have heard reports of products that are available to remove locks that are several years old. I am not sure about the authenticity of such products. From my vantage point, locking is a permanent process. Once the hair has locked permanently, the only way to get your hair back to a state where it can be combed again is by cutting all of your hair off. You truly have to be mentally ready to transform your hair into locks because it takes a lot of patience and understanding to transfer into this new style. Part of the understanding is realizing that the locks can take on a personality of their own. Some women find it devastating that they have to cut off all of their hair in order to come out of locking. Again, you have to be mentally ready. If I decide to cut my hair off, I will be ready to move on to the next hair process in this journey.

Chapter 9

The Rebirth of Me

I grew my locks long, wore the style for over six years, and I started to feel weighed down when I exercised and in my day-to-day activities. On Wednesday, April 23, 2008, I decided to cut my hair. When the beautician cut my hair, I felt as though a weight was lifted off me. I felt reborn. There was also a moment of sadness that I felt because I had long hair for so long that a part of me was missing when I cut my hair. However, since I am not afraid of trying new things, I was happy that I took the chance and did it.

After I got home excited about my new do, I got the look of uncertainty from my family, and at that point, I started to second-guess my decision and became upset by their reaction. I asked myself why I was so unnecessarily distraught over this. After a short period, they were used to it and thought it was very becoming on me.

I felt a number of emotions after I got my haircut. As one part of me was reborn, another part of me died as if I was in a state of mourning. I received many compliments everywhere I went, and I was told by several people the style suited me. I had to remember that *India Arie* reminds us that we are not our hair. She took a bold stance when she cut her hair completely off in protest because we put too much emphasis on hairstyle and texture. I understood the ideology of hair just being hair, and if it is cut, it can grow back which is no big deal, right? I do not know why I was uncomfortable with the thought of how other people would receive me with my new style. The bigger issue was why did I care? I began to realize that I still have a slight problem with being concerned about what people think. Nevertheless, I was happy about the change.

As I looked at myself again, I realized why I made the change. I recreated myself into something new and fresh. The new style gave me some pizzazz. Truly, it was a rebirth. Why was I upset? It is not as bad as I made it out to be, and my ill feelings were not based upon what I thought about myself but about what others perceived me to be. That is where I made my mistake. The style was not a mistake but my concern about what people thought of me was. We must realize that if we do not love ourselves, then who will. It is only hair, and I had to realize in this new transition that I am NOT my hair. There is so much more to me than what you see on the outside. I thank God for the realization of who I am on the inside.

Chapter 10

Moving on to the Future...

As you continue to contemplate what to do next with your hair, I hope that this book has provided you with some insight into that subject and will help you with your decision-making. As we all know, it is not easy to decide what to do next because of so many choices. People of African descent are very creative people. Some of us are trying to fit in with the corporate structure, staying connected with our roots, pleasing our family and friends, as well as pleasing ourselves. We do not want to step out of the "norm" and be ostracized but, at the same time, each of us knows what we want to do for ourselves. We need to look back into the past and grab hold of some of the hair styling techniques that were used back then. We should bring our many experiences and knowledge into the future to alleviate some of the hair problems that women experience today.

In relation to how we treat each other, we can be our own worst enemies when we are not supportive or positive toward one another. "Sistas" need to lift one another up and not tear one another down. Even if you have had negative experiences with some women, there are also women who are positive and help to boost your self-esteem. Traveling in positive circles is important and helps to keep the negative situations away as much as possible.

In our many experiences, we find that we have traveled down some roads in dealing with beauticians that are not "true professionals" and are unlicensed. The key is to investigate the beautician's background in order to find the right one for you. Also, it does help to use referrals to find a good beautician.

My experiences have taught me that life has taken me in many different directions, but each direction that I have taken has prepared me for the next level. I do not regret the choices that I have made in the past because I was predestined to try different things in order to appreciate what I have now. Each experience has the potential of having a positive outcome depending on how you look at it.

Having a positive mind, body, and soul has been critical for me in obtaining healthy hair. They can be obtained through using the right products for the hair, eating right, exercising, tapping into your spirituality with the understanding of God's word and having faith. Without these key elements, your overall health will suffer and that will definitely include the health of your hair.

In our day-to-day lives, we want our look to be professional and neat, and we need to try to make decisions that work in our best interest. Examine yourself and find out what you want to do with your hair because reinventing yourself is good. What will make you happy? Do you want to try something new? Make sure that you are doing what you do in order to preserve what God has blessed you with, and I hope that your trials, tribulations, and drama associated with having afro-textured hair become rare. Stay strong in the process and God Bless!

APPENDIX I.

Bonus Chapter:
History of Rastafarianism
and the Dreadlock

Let's get into the basics of the term "dread" according to the website www.dictionary.com that is associated with the "dreadlock." The meaning of the word "dread" is:

dread
v. dreaded, dreading, dreads
v. tr.
. To be in terror of.
. To anticipate with alarm, distaste, or reluctance: dreaded the long drive home.
. Archaic. To hold in awe or reverence.

v. intr.
To be very afraid.

n.
. Profound fear; terror.
. Fearful or distasteful anticipation. See Synonyms at fear.
. An object of fear, awe, or reverence.
. Archaic. Awe; reverence.

adj.
. Causing terror or fear: a dread disease.
. Inspiring awe: the dread presence of the headmaster.

The History of Rastafarian culture will connect us back to the very essence of the term dread and what dread actually means within the culture.

During the start of the Rastafarian culture when dreadlocks came about, some people feared them because they were thought to be scary and confrontational. The longer and more out of control the hair got the more fearful others were of them. The longer the hair grew the more "dreadful" they became hence the name "Dreadlock." They have a very interesting history dating back to the early 1900's. The dreadlock style is still popular to this day and people from different races wear the style.

Rastafarianism has a quasi-biblical base and is traced back to a Jamaican Black Nationalist named *Marcus Garvey*. He was instrumental in trying to organize the "Back to Africa Movement" due to the degradation that blacks endured as a result of slavery. Garvey founded the Universal Negro Improvement Association in the 1920's and preached about black self-empowerment and the abandonment of Eurocentric views. The movement was born when Garvey prophesied about a "black king being crowned." That king was *Ras Tafari Makonnen*, founder of the Rastafarian movement, who was crowned Emperor Haile Selassie 1 and was from Harer, Ethiopia. He claimed to be a direct descendent of King David and was proclaimed to be "King of Kings and Lord of Lords." The belief was that Emperor Haile Selassie 1 was the messiah who appeared to redeem blacks from white oppression. People were skeptical about the Rastafarian movement because it was thought that the Rasta's distorted the bible, smoked ganga, and drank alcohol. They had ongoing friction with the police because they were considered to be unruly.

The Dreadlock style is a twisted hairstyle that is virtually allowed to develop as the individual allows it to without much agitation. Dreadlocks have been compared to the lion's mane as a symbol of male strength hence as Rastas have stated, they are in the image of the "Lion of Judah." Rastafarians have cited the scripture Leviticus 21:15 as the justification for not cutting the hair.

Several organizations spawned from the Rastarian Movement. In the 1960's, adolescents saw the dreadlock as a way of rebelling from school and parental authority. The organization *Youth Black Faith* debated about whether or not to comb their hair. This was an issue that affected many because it was not acceptable to have unkempt hair. Not combing your hair meant you were trying to be antisocial. People who wore Dreadlocks were outcast so they wore them to invoke shock value.

There was also a community called the *"Bobo" Dread*. They lived in a compound and practiced many rituals. They lived about nine miles east of Kingston, Jamaica, wore tightly wrapped turbans, and long black/white robes. The leader was *Prince Emanuel*, and he was regarded as God. Other male members of the Bobo Dread were regarded as priests or prophets. The priests conducted services and the prophets were the voice of reason. In the compound, there was a guard at the gate protecting the community. Women and children were considered inferior to men. The children attended a school called "The Jerusalem School." I am not certain if the Bobo Dread still exist.

In the Rastafarian culture, it is estimated that there are 1,000,000 Rastafarians worldwide.

The history of Rastafarianism is indeed an interesting one. Being known for having dreadful hair can certainly make people feel defensive and less confident and cause low self-esteem. Equally, not understanding the reason why some people choose to keep their hair natural has been transcending into American culture causing negative terms to continue to perpetuate in American society.

The reason behind many of the natural styles being associated with negative terms is due to hatred, fear, and individuals not understanding each other. Natural styles have been looked upon as being a sign of strength and dignity and that is what brings about the fear in others. If people make you feel bad about your natural hair, then you will most likely change your hair to what makes others feel more comfortable. Your dignity has now diminished and you are no longer in control.

It is quite disturbing that negative terms have become a regular part of our vocabulary. For instance, the word *"nigger"* is so deeply rooted in African American culture. We have become very accustomed to the word and it is sometimes a part of the African American vocabulary used when addressing one another. It has been stated that our reasoning for allowing the word to permeate into our own vocabulary is so that we can take "control" over how the word is used. Whether we agree or disagree those same individuals using the word have stated that they are using it as a "term of endearment" turning it into a positive instead of a negative. Is it truly to use it as a term of endearment or is it merely a form of self-hatred continuing to manifest itself?

APPENDIX II.

Survey Raw Data

The following data was retrieved from the website form created to get a sense of how both women and men feel about the African American woman's hair. Questions numbered one through 15 were general questions and the additional questions asked were more specific to the particular hairstyle that the woman currently wears. The hairstyles surveyed were Braids/Cornrows, Chemically Processed (relaxer and curly perm), Locked, Other Natural Styles (not locked), Pressed, Weaved, or Wigs. Due to a technical difficulty, the result for pressed styles under the question pertaining to how a person feels about a particular style (like, dislike, unsure, no comment) came out to be inconclusive and is not represented in the tables.

Responses from the women

Questions 1 - 14

BC: Braids and Cornrows – 4 Responses	NS: Other Natural Styles – 10 Responses
CP: Chemical Processes – 41 Responses	PS: Pressed Styles – 3 Responses
WE: Weaves – 1 Response	WS: Wigs – 3 Responses
LS: Locked Styles – 4 Responses	

1. Where were you born?

	BC	CP	WE	LS	NS	PS	WS
USA	75%	98%	100%	100%	80%	67%	67%
Caribbean	25%	2%			20%	33%	33%

2. Where were you raised?

	BC	CP	WE	LS	NS	PS	WS
USA	75%	98%	100%	100%	80%	67%	67%
Caribbean	25%				20%	33%	33%
Other		2%					

3. What is your marital status?

	BC	CP	WE	LS	NS	PS	WS
Married	50%	46%		100%	50%	33%	67%
Single	50%	32%			10%		
Divorced		17%	100%		10%		
Widowed		5%			30%	67%	33%

4. If married, are you more or less inclined to wear your hair the way that your husband prefers?

	BC	CP	WE	LS	NS	PS	WS
More	25%	24%		25%	50%		
Less	25%	10%		25%	40%	33%	33%
N/A	50%	2%			10%		
Unans-wered		64%	100%	50%		67%	67%

5. How do you feel about relaxers?

	BC	CP	WE	LS	NS	PS	WS
Like	100%	83%	100%	75%	30%	67%	67%
Dislike		10%		25%	30%	33%	
Unsure		2%			30%		
No Comment		2%			10%		33%
Unans-wered		2%					

6. How do you feel about curly perms?

	BC	CP	WE	LS	NS	PS	WS
Like		46%			30%		
Dislike	50%	32%	100%	75%	40%	67%	
Unsure	25%	17%			20%		67%
No Comment	25%	5%		25%	10%	33%	33%

7. How do you feel about natural hairstyles?

	BC	CP	WE	LS	NS	PS	WS
Like	100%	76%	100%	100%	90%	100%	67%
Dislike		7%					
Unsure		15%			10%		
No Comment		2%					33%

8. How do you feel about hair extensions?

	BC	CP	WE	LS	NS	PS	WS
Like	50%	39%	100%	50%	60%	33%	67%
Dislike	50%	29%		25%	20%	67%	
Unsure		22%			20%		33%
No Comment		10%		25%			

9. How do you feel about braids/cornrows?

	BC	CP	WE	LS	NS	PS	WS
Like	100%	80%	100%	100%	60%	100%	67%
Dislike					30%		
Unsure		7%			10%		33%
No Comment		10%					
Un-answered		3%					

10. How do you feel about wigs?

	BC	CP	WE	LS	NS	PS	WS
Like	75%	46%		25%	70%		100%
Dislike	25%	25%		50%	10%	67%	
Unsure		23%	100%	25%	10%	33%	
No Comment		10%			10%		

11. How do you feel about locks?

	BC	CP	WE	LS	NS	PS	WS
Like	75%	60%		100%	60%	33%	67%
Dislike		20%			30%	33%	33%
Unsure	25%	13%	100%		10%	33%	
No Comment		8%					

12. Which way do you prefer to wear your hair most of the time?

	BC	CP	WE	LS	NS	PS	WS
Chemical Processed	75%	75%					67%
Natural	25%	8%			90%	67%	
Weave		5%	100%		10%		33%
Braids/ Cornrows		13%					
Locks				100%			
Unanswered						33%	

13. If you go to a professional salon, how do you feel after getting your hair done?

	BC	CP	WE	LS	NS	PS	WS
Very Good	75%	49%		25%	60%		67%
Good	25%	32%	100%	25%	10%		
Alright		15%		25%	10%	67%	
Fair		2%			10%		
N/A				25%	10%	33%	33%

14. Do you find yourself changing you hair to keep up with the latest fads?

	BC	CP	WE	LS	NS	PS	WS
Yes	25%	17%	100%	25%	10%	33%	33%
No	75%	83%		75%	90%	67%	67%

BRAIDS/CORNROWS QUESTIONS #15-24

15. Do you have your hair braided or cornrowed in a professional or non-professional location?

Professional	50%
Non-Professional	50%

16. How often do you go for your hair to be re-done?

Every 8 weeks	25%
Every 6 weeks	25%
Every 4 weeks	
Other-Every 2 weeks	25%
Other-No Comment	25%

17. How long does the style last?

Four months	
Three months	
Two Months	25%
Other- 3 days	25%
Other – 2 weeks	25%
Unanswered	25%

18. Are you satisfied with the length of time that your hairstyle lasts?

Yes	50%
No	50%

19. Have you experienced any extreme breakage and/or baldness from the braiding or any other problems from braiding?

Yes	75%
No	25%

20. Have you had any breakage around the hairline due to the braids or cornrows?

Yes	50%
No	50%

21. Do you prefer braids or cornrows?

Braids	50%
Cornrows	50%

22. Have you experienced any negative comments at your place of employment due to your braids/cornrows?

Yes	
No	100%

23. Why do you choose to wear braids or cornrows?

I like the style	
Convenience	25%
Last long	25%
Other	50%

24. How many years have you worn braids/ cornrows?

15 years or more	
10 to 15 years	
5 to 10 years	25%
1 to 5 years	50%
Unanswered	25%

CHEMICAL PROCESS QUESTIONS #15-23

15. Which of the following forms of chemical processing do you currently use?

Relaxers	93%
Curly Perm	7%

16. Do you prefer....

Relaxer	80%
Curly Perm	7%
Both	13%

17. Do you go to a professional salon or do you do your own processing?

Go to a Salon	68%
Do my own	27%
Unanswered	5%

18. How often do you have to have touch-ups on your process?

Every 8 weeks	37%
Every 6 weeks	32%
Every 4 weeks	10%
Other – Every 10 weeks	22%

19. Are you satisfied with the length of time that you hair lasts after you have it done?

Yes	78%
No	22%

20. Have you experienced any extreme breakages and/or baldness as a result of the chemical?

Yes	22%
No	78%

21. Did you experience any other problems from the use of chemicals?

Yes	33%
No	67%

22. Have you ever had to cut off all of your hair to "start over" after using a chemical?

Yes	22%
No	78%

23. How many years have you worn your hair in a chemical process?

More than 15 years	71%
11 to 15 years	22%
6 to 10 years	2%
1 to 5 years	
Less than 1 year	5%

LOCKS QUESTIONS #15-22

15. Do you go to a professional salon or a non-professional location to have your locks re-twisted?

Professional Salon	50%
Non-Professional Location	50%

16. How often do you go to get your locks re-twisted?

Every 8 weeks	25%
Every 6 weeks	25%
Every 4 weeks	
Other	50%

17. Are you satisfied with the length of time that your hair lasts?

Yes	75%
No	25%

18. Have you ever experienced any extreme breakage and/or baldness from the locking process?

Yes	
No	100%

19. Did you experience any other problems from the twisting process?

Yes	25%
No	75%

20. What are you wearing your hair in a locked style?

I like the style	25%
Convenience	
Keeps your hair healthy	
To stay connected with your race	
Other	75%

21. Have you experienced any negative comments at your place of employment due to your locks?

Yes	25%
No	75%

22. How many years have you worn locks?

More than 15 years	
11 to 15 years	
6 to 10 years	25%
1 to 5 years	75%
Less than 1 year	

OTHER NATURAL STYLES QUESTIONS #15-22

15. Have you ever felt ashamed about your hair being in its natural state?

Yes	10%
No	90%

16. Have you ever been made to feel bad about your hair by someone else?

Yes	50%
No	50%

17. Have you ever been caught up with the "good" hair "bad" hair syndrome?

Yes	70%
No	30%

18. Have you ever felt that your hair was too difficult to deal with in its natural state?

Yes	50%
No	50%

19. Have you ever felt that you didn't have enough preparation time to deal with you hair in its natural state?

Yes	20%
No	70%
Unanswered	10%

20. Are you comfortable with your hair texture?

Yes	90%
No	10%

21. Is there anything that you would change about your hair texture?

Yes	30%
No	70%

22. How many years have you worn your hair in its natural state?

More than 15 years	40%
11 to 15 years	10%
6 to 10 years	20%
1 to 5 years	30%
Less than 1 year	

PRESSED HAIR STYLES QUESTIONS #15-21

15. How often do you have your hair pressed?

Every 8 weeks	
Every 6 weeks	
Every 4 weeks	
Other-Every 3 weeks	67%
Other-No Comment	
Unanswered	33%

16. Do you go to a professional salon to have your hair pressed or do you do your own hair?

Professional Salon	67%
Do my own hair	33%

17. How long does the "style" last you after either going to a salon or doing your own hair?

One month	
Three weeks	33%
Two weeks	
One week	67%
Other	

18. Are you satisfied with the length of time that your hair lasts you after going to a salon or doing your own hair?

Yes	67%
No	33%

19. Have you ever experienced any breakage and/or baldness from having your hair pressed?

Yes	33%
No	67%

20. Have you experienced any other problems from having your hair pressed?

Yes	
No	100%

21. How many years have you worn your hair pressed?

More than 15 years	33%
11 to 15 years	33%
6 to 10 years	33%
1 to 5 years	
Less than 1 year	

WEAVE/HAIR EXTENSIONS QUESTIONS #15-21

15. Do you have your extensions done at a professional salon?

Yes	100%
No	

16. How often do you go to have the extensions re-done?

Every 8 weeks	100%
Every 6 weeks	
Every 4 weeks	
Other	

17. Are you satisfied with the length of time that your hair lasts?

Yes	100%
No	

18. Have you ever experienced any extreme breakage and/or baldness from the extensions?

Yes	
No	100%

19. Did you experience any other problems from the extensions?

Yes	100%
No	

20. Why do you choose to wear hair extensions?

I like the style	
I like the fullness and length that it gives	
Protects/preserves my own hair	
Other	100%

21. How many years have you worn hair extensions?

More than 15 years	
11 to 15 years	
6 to 10 years	
1 to 5 years	100%
Less than 1 year	

WIGS QUESTIONS #15-21

15. How often do you have to purchase a new wig?

Every 8 weeks	33%
Every 6 weeks	
Every 4 weeks	67%
Other	

16. Are you satisfied with the length of time that your wig lasts you after you purchase a new one?

Yes	100%
No	

17. Have you experienced any breakage and/or baldness around the hairline from the wig?

Yes	33%
No	67%

18. Did you experience any other problems from the wig?

Irritation and/or redness	
Itchiness and/or allergic reaction	
Not fitting properly	33%
Unanswered	67%

19. Why have you worn a wig?

Convenience	67%
Like the styles	
Easy to deal with	
Unanswered	33%

20. Has wearing a wig been cost effective for you?

Yes	67%
No	33%

21. How many years have you worn wigs?

More than 15 years	33%
11 to 15 years	
6 to 10 years	
1 to 5 years	33%
Less than 1 year	33%

Responses from the men
QUESTIONS #1-10
15 Responses

1. How do you feel about your wife or girlfriend's hair?

Like	80%
Dislike	7%
Unsure	13%

2. Do you prefer natural or chemically processed styles?

Natural	67%
Chemical	13%
Both	20%

3. What type of style do you like her to wear?

Long	33%
Short	13%
The way she likes	13%
Braids	20%
Twists	7%
Afro	13%

4. What are you thoughts about beauty salons?

Like	47%
Dislike	7%
Too much money	20%
Too much time	13%
Too many	7%

5. Has your wife or girlfriend spent a lot of time at the beauty salon on any given appointment?

Yes	60%
No	33%
Unknown	7%

6. What do you think about the cost that she pays at the beauty salon?

Too much money	33%
O.K. with the cost	27%
Unknown	33%
N/A	7%

7. Approximately how long does it take your wife or girlfriend to get her hair done at the beauty salon?

6-8 hours	13%
3-5 hours	20%
2-2 ½ hours	20%
½ to 1 ½ hours	13%
Unknown	27%
No Answer	7%

8. How long does it take for her to get her hair ready if you are going out on a date?

Too long	7%
1-2 hours	27%
Less than ½ hour	60%
Unknown	7%

9. Does she take too much time to prepare for a date or are you o.k. with the time it takes her?

Yes	67%
No	33%

10. If you could choose a style for her, what style would it be?

Long	27%
Straight	7%
Short	20%
Variety	13%
Braids	13%
Afro	7%
Twists	7%
Unknown	7%

APPENDIX III.

Survey Participant Comments

From the individuals who responded to the Braids and Cornrows survey...

"Getting my hair permed allows me to maintain a better style for a longer period than the others listed."

"At times, it is more affordable to get my hair cornrowed rather than permed and styled at a professional salon. Whatever style I wear in my hair is based on what I can afford in that given week."

"As stated, my style of preference is normally a perm and style, however, since there are times when I cannot afford a professional salon visit, I go to a non-professional establishment to get the braids. Although I do realize that it is damaging to my hair. I guess vanity, the desire to look presentable outweighs logic at times. Thank you for allowing me to participate."

"I experienced extreme breakage when I went swimming and I went to comb my hair and it was so nappy that it kept breaking. I want my hair longer."

"Chemical processing causes breakage when I let the new growth go for more than 6 weeks."

"I choose to wear braids because they are convenient and long lasting."

From the individuals who responded to the Chemically Processed survey...

"Had a beautician once to over process my hair causing it to thin out making it not manageable or able to hold any style. This is also someone who makes her own products and specializes in natural, multiethnic hair and styles."

"I have cut all my hair off by choice once and gone natural for about a year or two and then decided to allow my hair to grow back out and get a perm. I just didn't feel the natural look was a complimentary look for myself. One day, I may try it again, because my hair was extremely healthy and thicker upon letting it grow back out."

"I have used hair dye and it made my hair very dry."

"Usually 8 weeks or more my hair is very fine so I try not to over process it"

"For many years, I wore my hair in its natural state and changed as I do from time to time for something different. This perm is also a phase! And this too shall pass!"

"I know in my case, my hair style is based on the conservative job that I have. Sometimes I think we adjust not necessarily to our preference but with what we think may enhance our career."

"Impatience with process of going natural"

"A rash on my neckline, from relaxer cream touching the skin"

"I tried to go natural once but I did not like the twilight period between go natural and having the perm. I guess I didn't give myself enough time and hope to go natural in the future."

"I prefer to wear my hair in braids because it is comfortable and the weave and extensions can fall out at school or other places that is if you don't put it in right. I like the relaxers and curly perms but not all the time. I usually wear braids or cornrows or out and the locks, well, that could be mom's style but not mine because you can do lots of things with it but the catch is if you pull it out or take it out your hair will fall out otherwise no hair a.k.a. one at all!!!"

"Other problems….Dryness (leading to other problems), brittle, lacking luster, dependency to chemicals & costly."

"I prefer to wear my hair weaved -- You always have a nice hair style when you wear a wig – weather does not affect the style."

"After a new relaxer touch-up, my scalp is dry."

"I prefer to wear my hair: Chemical Processed—I like the long, straight look."

"I prefer to wear my hair: Chemical Processed—I like the way it looks on me."

"I prefer to wear my hair: Braids—I don't have to comb it."

"I prefer to wear my hair: Chemical Processed—Easier for me."

"If my hair is not in a natural style, I prefer having a perm because it makes my hair more manageable and look nice. I had a natural for about 2 years and just didn't feel that it looked as good on me as it does when my hair is relaxed. As well as it was difficult for me to find a hair care provider that would help me to take care of it, since I had relocated to a new city. I would not rule out going back to a natural look in the future."

I only experienced problems, when I attempted to maintain my hair on my own."

"Other problems: Scalp burns"

"I prefer to wear my hair: Chemical Processed—during the summer only because of the humidity."

"I like locks that are maintained. I do not like dreadlocks. I've been told that dreadlocks are worn by African witch doctors. The dreadlocks have a dark origin."

"My hair is chemically processed. I like simple styles. I thank God for beauty salons. I try not to spend too much time in beauty salons. It takes me about 1 hour at the beauty salon. I shampoo my own hair. It takes me 20 minutes to get my hair together. The money I pay to beauty salons is too high. I like simple styles."

"I prefer to wear my hair: Chemical Processed -- It is easier to keep neat and professional looking."

"I prefer to wear my hair: Natural—it's easier."

"I have had some breakage at various times. I'm not sure what the cause was."

"We have come a long way with what the black women do to their hair. Getting better and beautiful."

"I would have liked to expand on question #5. Although I dislike perms, I do like how they make my hair look versus any other style."

From the individuals who responded to the Weave/Hair Extensions survey...

"Have you experienced problems: Itchy scalp, and my hair not remaining in place over the top of the extensions sewn in place."

"I like the style, I like the fullness and length that it gives, and it protects and preserves my own hair."

From the individuals who responded to the Locks survey...

"Do not want chemical and feel that weaves should only be used when necessary."

"I no longer want to use chemicals and I no longer want to cut my hair."

"I prefer to wear my hair: Locks—I like the look and It is easy to care for."

"I wear my hair in this style for all of the reasons given, i.e. I like the style, convenience, keeps my hair healthy, and helps me to stay connected to my race."

"I prefer to wear my hair: Locks—easy, natural."

"One of my twists in the back is becoming smaller at the root. Maybe it's because of being twisted too tightly."

"Why are you wearing locks: For all of the above, i.e. I like the style, convenience, keeps my hair healthy, and helps me to stay connected to my race."

From the individuals who responded to the Other Natural Styles survey...

"I would like for my hair to have less frizz."

"I like my hair...being bi-racial gives a certain jazzy quality that complements my personality."

"I wish I had mom's hair. Her hair was all the way down to her bottom because of our (partial) Indian heritage on mom's side. Dad was of pure African heritage."

"I like natural because of the ease of care, less damage than perms. I wish it was thicker right after it is washed. I actually have fine hair. I use a semi-permanent hair color. The color is okay, it's black and no it hasn't damaged my hair as far as I can tell. Good survey. I cut off my hair in December because every time I received a relaxer it burned no matter the strength."

From the individuals who responded to the Pressed Styles survey...

"From frequently coloring my hair over 20 years, I have had hair breakage about 3 or 4 times. I corrected the problem by using different products to strengthen and moisturize my hair."

"I prefer to wear my hair: Weave—Low maintenance."

"I have my hair done: Every weekend."

From the individuals who responded to the Wigs survey...

"I prefer to wear my hair: Weave—It's convenient."

"I prefer to wear my hair: Chemical Processed—manageable."

Men's Survey Comments

Question 1 Responses – How do you feel about your wife or girlfriend's hair?

Well, I like it because it's easy. She can get dressed faster and doesn't have to use rollers.
It should be done at all times whether you are going anywhere or not.
It looks good.
I am happy with it.
I love to play with it. Run my fingers thru it and pull at it when we make love.
I like the way it looks on her.
I wish she would let it grow.
She's never satisfied with it. It drives me crazy!
I'd rather she wear it natural because her hair is thicker than the "permed" out look.
I'm fine with it.
Happy for her.
Good.
I like when her she has her hair straightened.
She has a short afro and it is nice to me.
She takes good care of it. I like it.

Question 2 Responses - Do you prefer natural or chemically processed styles?

Natural
I really like the natural hairstyles. I prefer natural if your hair is good. If you have bad hair, you may need a chemical.
Processed
Natural
No preference because I don't know the difference between them. Does it look good is all I care about.
Both
Natural
Natural with no add-in hair (if you know what I mean)
Natural
It doesn't matter.
Natural
Natural
I prefer chemicals.
I like natural styles.
I prefer the natural styles.

Question 3 Responses - What type of style do you like her to wear?

Hanging down.
I like the mushroom style, the wrap style, the bang style and the bun style.
Short
Hair out, long.
It doesn't matter as long as her hair style makes her feel attractive and sexy.
Microbraids
A short style.
Natural twist or pulled straight back.
Braids, afro puffs, anything natural.
Whatever she likes.
Afro
Long
I like braids, doobie, straight hair.
I would prefer her to keep her hair as it is.
Straight down; non-curled.

Question 4 Responses – What are your thoughts about beauty salons?

Too much money. Too much time spent.
I like beauty salons because they have a choice of different styles that you may want to see your lady in.
They are too time consuming
They are fine
If they can find a way to not keep my wife half of the day, I would love them more.
They are a female version of a barbershop.
Great idea.
It's o.k. Don't like all the gossip
Beauty is without a doubt within. God made us "all" beautiful in our own unique way. Make-up doesn't help if the inside is hideous.
I'm cool with them.
Prices are too high
Like
I think they overcharge for what people want to have done.
They are good. If it makes my baby feel good then go ahead
There are too many of them now.

Question 5 Responses – Has your wife or girlfriend spent a lot of time at the beauty salon on any given appointment?

Yes!!!!
No, she doesn't go.
Yes.
Yes. Several hours
Yes.
Yes.
Yes.
Yes, sometimes 6 to 7 hours. That's too much time.
Nope.
Unknown
Yes.
Yes.
No.
No.
No. She does hair and takes care of hers

Question 6 Responses – Approximately how long does it take your wife or girlfriend to get her hair done at the beauty salon?

5 hours
N/A
1 ½ to 2 hours
3 hours
Depending on the style and day she goes, she has spent up to 8 hours there.
3-6 hours
About 1 hour
On average 2 ½ hours
Minus ½ a second, she doesn't go.
Unknown
Don't know
3 hours
1 ½ to 2 hours
About an hour
1 ½ hours

Question 7 Responses – How long does it take for her to get her hair ready if you are going out on a date?

1 hour or so
About a half hour
15 minutes
45 minutes
30-45 minutes
10-15 minutes
20 minutes
1 to 2 hours
10 minutes
Unknown
Too long
1 hour
1 to 1 ½ hours. She takes a long time.
About 30 minutes
Less than 15 minutes

Question 8 Responses – Does she take too much time to prepare for a date or are you o.k. with the time it takes her?

I want it to go faster.
I am o.k. with the time it takes her because I would rather her look nice instead of rushing. I don't care how long it takes. She should start a couple of hours ahead of time. I don't want her looking any kind of way.
O.K. she's gotten better
I have come to expect it so I am o.k. with it
I am o.k. with it.
It is o.k.
No
Takes too long for me because she's never satisfied with her hair no matter what she does to it.
I'm o.k. with it.
It doesn't bother me.
Too long
No
I am o.k. with the time that it takes.
I'm o.k. with the time.
I'm o.k. with the time it takes her.

Question 9 Responses – What do you think about the cost that she pays at the beauty salon?

Too much money
N/A
Modest
The cost is fine.
Too much
I don't know how much she spends on hair
No
Somewhat on the overpriced end
Love it $0
Unknown
Too high
No problem
I think generally they overcharge, however she doesn't have to pay because she works there.
Cost is fine
N/A

Question 10 Responses – If you could choose a style for her, what style would it be?

Hanging down; hair flowing
I would like to see her in some braids.
Short and curly
Nice, natural and long
My wife always ask me how I would like to see her hair styles so we switch up sometimes long sometimes in braids others short. She is very flexible. The only thing I ask her not to do is any buns. I guess I am pretty lucky now that I think about my answer to this question.
Microbraids
Afro
Natural curls or twisted style
On any given day be versatile...
Unknown
Bald
Long
Just straight; laying down
Short afro
Straight wild; non-curled look but is done

APPENDIX IV.

Photo Montage

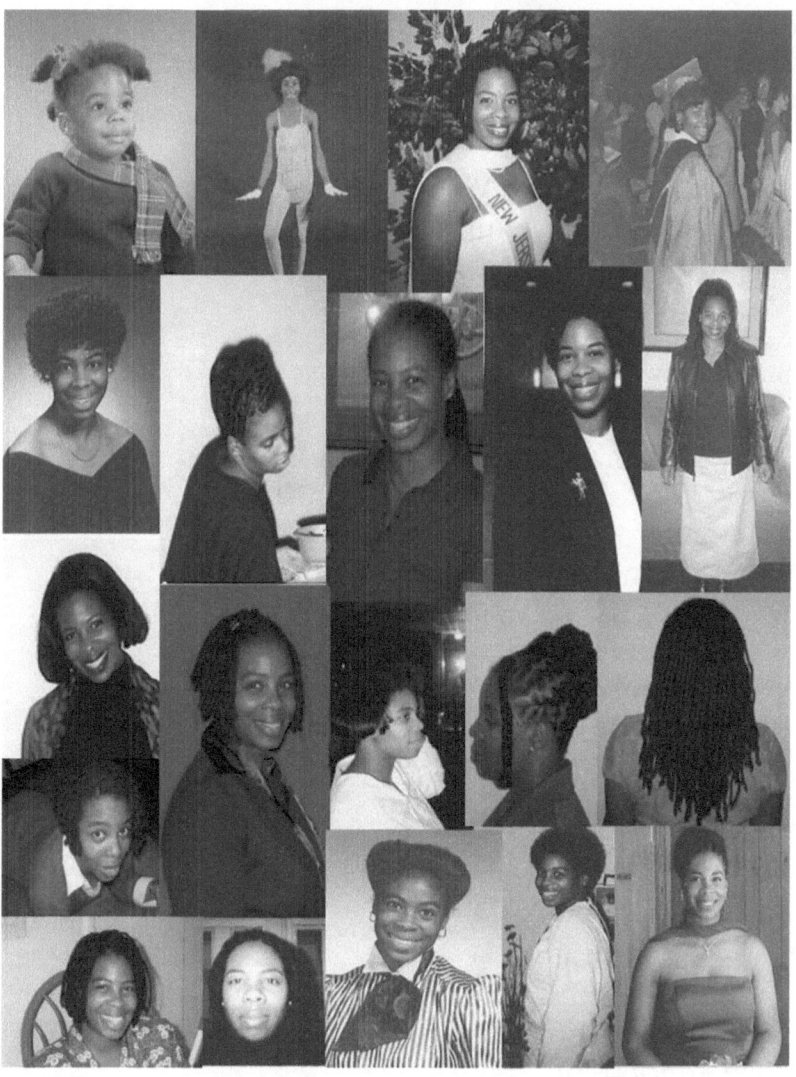

APPENDIX V.

Website Addresses

Below are some websites that may be useful to you. I hope you enjoy them!

Natural Hair Care Websites
www.adoptn.org/hair.html
www.afrohair.com
www.allbraiding.com
www.blackbeautyandhair.com
www.blackhairdvd.com
www.blackhairmedia.com/hairstyles
www.blackhairplanet.com
http://blackhairtalk.proboards30.com
www.going-natural.com
www.hisandher.com
www.nappturality.com
www.treasuredlocks.com/blhacafa.html

Skin and Hair Products Websites
www.blackstylists.com
www.bobsaone.org
www.carolsdaughter.com
www.drmaclin.com
www.especiallyyours.com
www.jazma.com
www.locksandlinks.com
www.lusterproducts.com
www.motionshair.com
www.ultrablackhair.com

Salons
www.salonsofamerica.com
www.universalsalons.com

Media and News Sites
www.blacknews.com/directory/black_african_
american_hair.shtml
www.hypehair.com
www.naturalhairdigest.com
www.sizta2sizta.com
www.sophicatesblackhairstyles.com

BIBLIOGRAPHY

<u>Books</u>

Ahkell, Jah. *Rasta: Emperor Haile Selassie and the Rastafarians*, Frontline Distribution, 1997.

Barrett, Sr., Leonard E. *The Rastafarians*, Beacon Press, 1997.

Barrow, Steve. *The Rough Guide to Reggae*, Rough Guides, Ltd., 1997.

Brittenum Bonner, Lonnice. *Good Hair.* Random House, Inc. 1994.

Campbell, Horace. *Rasta and Resistance: From Marcus Garvey to Walter Rodney.* Africa World Press, Inc., 1987.

Chevannes, Barry. *Rastafari: Roots and Ideology.* Syracuse University Press, 1994.

Evans, Nekhena. *Hairlocking Everything you need to know.* A&B Publishers Group. 1999.

Hausman, Gerald. *The Kebra Negast – The Book of Rastafarian Faith from Ethiopia and Jamaica.* St. Martin's Press, 1997.

Serikali, Kumasi. *Hair Locking A Guide for the Amateur Locktician.* Epic Press. 2000.

Shamboosie. *Beautiful Black Hair.* Amber Communications Group, Inc., 2002.

Websites

Bellis, Mary. *Madame C.J. Walker.* New York Times Company 2009. http://inventors.about.com/od/wstartinventors/a/MadameWalker.htm

Chevannes, Barry. *The Bobo Dread.* Renzo Taddei 2001. http://www.tc.columbia.edu/centers/cifas/Drugsandsociety/analyses/chevannes1.html

"dread." © *Encyclopædia Britannica, Inc..* Encyclopædia Britannica, Inc. 25 Sep. 2009. http://dictionary.reference.com/browse/dread

Hair Follicle. n.d. http://en.wikipedia.org/wiki/Hair_follicle.

Homiak, Dr. Jake. *Dread History: The African Diaspora, Ethianopianism, and Rastafari.* Smithsonian Center for Education and Museum Studies n.d. http://www.smithsonianeducation.org/migrations/rasta/rasta.html

McClain, Cassia. *The Truth about Hair Relaxers.* Dr. Loren Pickart 2008. http://www.skinbiology.com/truthabouthairrelaxers.html

USDA Center for Nutrition Policy and Promotion. Food Pyramid. 2009. http://www.mypyramid.gov

MY THANKS TO YOU

Thank you so very much for purchasing my book. I am truly grateful to you who are a part of making this project a success. I hope that it was inspiring to you. May God richly, and immensely bless you!

Upcoming Book Projects...

Please go to website address: www.writingsbyasj.com for more details on my upcoming book projects.
I invite you to give me your comments on this book project. You can reach me at nomorehairdrama@writingsbyasj.com.

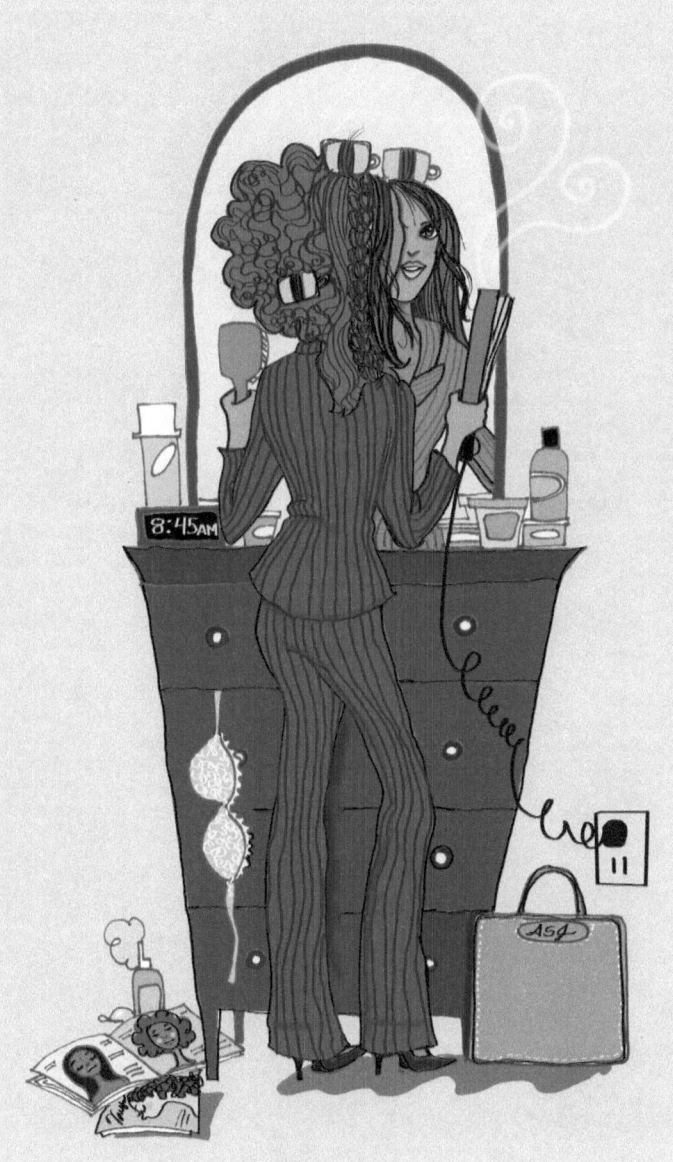

www.ingramcontent.com/pod-product-compliance
Lightning Source LLC
Chambersburg PA
CBHW061304280526
45784CB00002B/887